The Assessment and Treatment of Children Who Abuse Animals

Kenneth Shapiro • Mary Lou Randour
Susan Krinsk • Joann L. Wolf

The Assessment and Treatment of Children Who Abuse Animals

The AniCare Child Approach

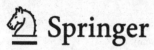 Springer

Kenneth Shapiro
Animals and Society Institute, Inc.
Washington Grove, MD
USA

Susan Krinsk
Child Protective Center
Sarasota, FL
USA

Mary Lou Randour
Animal Welfare Institute
Washington, DC
USA

Joann L. Wolf
Put-in-Bay, OH
USA

Previous editions originally been published by the society under the title: "AniCare Child: An Assessment and Treatment Approach for Children who Abuse Animals" (2006, 2002).

ISBN 978-3-319-01088-5   ISBN 978-3-319-01089-2   (eBook)
DOI 10.1007/978-3-319-01089-2
Springer Cham Heidelberg New York Dordrecht London

Library of Congress Control Number: 2013948395

Springer is part of Springer Science+Business Media (www.springer.com)

The Assessment and Treatment of Children Who Abuse Animals

The AniCare Child Approach

by

Kenneth Shapiro, PhD, ABPP, Mary Lou Randour, PhD
Susan Krinsk, LMHC, Joanne L. Wolf, MA, CAC

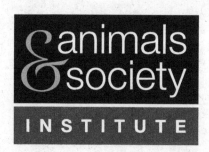

A project of the Animals and Society Institute
3rd Edition 2013; 2nd Edition 2006; 1st Edition 2002

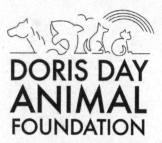

The Animals and Society Institute thanks the
Doris Day Animal Foundation for its generous support.

AniCare is a registered service mark of the Animals and Society Institute

Using *AniCare Child*

AniCare Child offers an approach for assessing and treating childhood cruelty to nonhuman animals (hereafter animals) and is designed for two audiences. The primary audience consists of mental health professionals working with children in agencies, domestic violence organizations, hospitals, schools, and private practice. Secondarily, *AniCare Child* will be useful to other professionals who work with children and their families—day-care providers, social service workers, probation department and other law enforcement officials, teachers, clergy, animal control and humane society personnel, and veterinarians.

For ease of use and to suit the different needs of potential users, *AniCare Child* is divided into three sections: Theory, Assessment, and Treatment. Some users, such as day-care providers or teachers, might find the assessment section most useful but will refer children to a mental health professional for treatment. All three sections of *AniCare Child* will be useful to mental health professionals. *AniCare Child* can be used in a number of ways. It can be the major focus of treatment with children who are referred—either by the courts, schools, or their parents—specifically for animal abuse. In other cases, the clinician may determine that a child, referred to treatment for some other reason, mistreats animals. In these instances, *AniCare Child* may supplement the ongoing treatment. In all cases, *AniCare Child* should be used within the framework of a comprehensive assessment and treatment plan.

Although we developed *AniCare Child* for use in an individual counseling setting, most of the assessment and interventions are readily adaptable for working with groups. With the further recognition of the need for the treatment of juveniles who abuse animals, in future it could become more practical to provide intervention in a group setting. Particularly when dealing, as in this clinical population, with socially unacceptable behavior, the dynamics of a group of peers can be an important vehicle for change.

This third edition of *AniCare Child* (2013) reflects the collective experience garnered from the presentation of 65 AniCare Child and AniCare Adult workshops in 23 states. Since 2008, we have also offered an online course on the AniCare approach through the School of Social Work at Arizona State University. (The course is one of a series of two leading to a certificate in the treatment of animal abuse.) In addition to the direct contributions of the individuals listed in the Acknowledgments, we have gained from the suggestions of the 18 certified AniCare trainers who colead workshops.

As a result of these experiences and input from these individuals, the third edition contains much new material. Note the following major changes:

- Theory section with emphasis on attachment theory
- Integration of the "Working with Parents" section into the Treatment section
- Material on trauma-informed narrative
- Updated research findings on witnessing abuse

In addition, the following supplemental materials and services are available from the Animals and Society Institute (ASI):

- The AniCare Demonstration DVD illustrates some of the assessment instruments and interventions in the handbook through role-played interviews. References to relevant segments are provided throughout the text.
- The AniCare Workshop DVD is a tape of major segments of a recent workshop (September 2011), emphasizing the conceptual material.
- *The AniCare Child Companion Workbook* provides homework and exercises for clients.
- *The AniCare Model for Treatment of Animal Abuse*, a handbook and accompanying demonstration DVD for adults who abuse animals, may be useful, particularly when assessing and treating juveniles 16 years and older.
- AniCareAction is a listserv that allows therapists and other interested parties to share their experiences with the AniCare Approach: http://groups.yahoo.com/group/anicareaction

To obtain these helpful supplemental materials, information about consultation on cases involving AniCare, training to become a trainer in the AniCare approach, and an opportunity to participate in an evaluation study, contact us at:

2512 Carpenter Road, Suite 202-A Ann Arbor, MI 48108–1188

by telephone at:
734-677-9240
or e-mail at
ken.shapiro@animalsandsociety.org

or visit our website at:
http://www.animalsandsociety.org/pages/anicare

Acknowledgments

Thanks to major funding from the Kenneth A. Scott Charitable Trust and additional grants from the Claire Giannini Fund, the Max Factor Family Fund, and the Frederick H. Leonhardt Foundation, we are pleased to present the third edition of *AniCare Child*.

We also would like to thank the following therapists and researchers who have contributed generously to sections of the revision: Aubrey Fine, Maya Gupta, Antonia Henderson, Risa Mandell, Kate Nicoll, Nancy Parrish, and Sharon Scott. Special thanks to Jill Howard Church for copyediting, Kate Brindle for formatting, and Jojo Shapiro for artwork.

Contents

1.1 The Need

There are treatments available for children with a wide variety of problems, including behavioral disorders, fire-setting, and other syndromes such as anxiety disorders, depression, sleep problems, and encopresis. Although juvenile animal abuse is far too common, and has long-standing and multiple negative consequences for the child and society, until the publication of *AniCare Adult* in 1998 and the first edition of *AniCare Child* in 2002, there was no treatment approach with an exclusive focus on juvenile animal abuse. *AniCare Child* filled that gap by providing specific and reliable treatment approaches for children who abuse animals.

1.2 Development of AniCare Child

The development of *AniCare Child* is based on clinical experience, a review of effective treatments for children that are relevant to this topic, and consultation with and review by other experts. Two of the coauthors of *AniCare Child*, who have considerable experience working with children with behavioral problems such as animal abuse and provided detailed clinical insight, are Susan Krinsk, LMHC of the Child Protection Center of Sarasota, Florida, and Joey Wolf, M.A., formerly Director of the Aurora Center for Treatment in Aurora, Colorado. The other coauthor, Mary Lou Randour, Ph.D., also coauthored *AniCare Adult*.

In addition to the coauthors, a number of others helped develop *AniCare Child*. Other contributors to *AniCare Child* provided valuable feedback, read early drafts, and offered important clinical and theoretical insights: Frank Ascione, Ph.D.; Edith A. Bennett, Ph.D.; Barbara Boat, Ph.D.; Peter Campos, Ph.D.; Deborah Matthews, Ph.D.; and Richard Ruth, Ph.D.

Undertaken by Kenneth Shapiro, the third edition applies the collected experience of several AniCare-certified trainers who have conducted 65 workshops in 23 states. *AniCare Child* encompasses several theoretical perspectives—attachment

K. Shapiro et al., *The Assessment and Treatment of Children Who Abuse Animals*, DOI 10.1007/978-3-319-01089-2_1, © Springer International Publishing Switzerland 2014

theory, cognitive behaviorism and trauma-informed personal narrative, and psychodynamic theory.

Although clinicians are generally trained in a particular theoretical orientation, many clinicians adopt an eclectic approach, borrowing from other perspectives as needed. The interventions of *AniCare Child*, which draw from numerous sources, are useful for clinicians of varied theoretical backgrounds.

1.3 Background

Juvenile crime statistics portray a disturbing trend in the last several decades. Youth violence began to increase in the 1960s, and while it remained high, it also showed relative stability until the mid-1980s. It then began to increase steadily, shooting up dramatically in 1993, and then slowly declining to the (still high) rate of the 1980s.

Although the troubling spike of youth violence in 1993 has abated, it remains the second leading cause of death for youth between the ages of 10 and 24 (Centers for Disease Control, 2010). Additionally, much attention is now being given "low-level aggression," which includes such antisocial acts as verbal insults, pushing and shoving, violating rules, and theft (Moeller, 2001). Researchers have documented the negative impact of bullying (Hilton, Anngela-Cole, & Wakita, 2010). Some writers contend that engaging in low-level aggressive behaviors encourages the commission of more violent acts (Goldstein, 1999; Toby, 1995). Data from the large-scale longitudinal Pittsburgh Youth Study (Loeber et al., 1993) suggest multiple developmental pathways from low-level aggression to more serious acts of delinquency. Youth violence at all levels, from bullying to school shootings, remains a troubling problem for society.

One significant manifestation of youth violence is juvenile animal abuse. It has been reported that many youths involved with US school shootings had engaged in various forms of animal abuse (Miner, 1999; Verlinden, Hersen, & Thomas, 2000). According to the FBI, in almost all cases, serial killers had histories of animal abuse in their youth (Lockwood & Hodge, 1998).

In addition to these dramatic examples, an accumulating body of psychological and other social science research provides substantial evidence for a link between animal abuse and human violence. Frick et al. (1993) identified animal abuse as one of the earliest-onset symptoms of conduct disorder, a diagnosis characterized by repetitive violation of social norms or others' rights and a prerequisite for an adult diagnosis of Antisocial Personality Disorder. Research studies comparing incarcerated adult males to noncriminal men have found a significant association between animal cruelty in childhood and serious, recurrent aggression against people as an adult (Felthous & Kellert, 1987). Another comprehensive study showed that adult men convicted of animal abuse were much more likely to have perpetrated violence against humans, committed crimes against property, and been arrested for substance abuse or drunk and disorderly charges when compared to similar men who had no animal abuse convictions (Luke, Arluke, & Levin, 1997). Similarly, a three-year study by the Chicago Police Department found that 65 % of people arrested for animal abuse crimes were also arrested for violent crimes against people (Degenhardt, 2004). In the Pittsburgh Youth Study described above, physical aggression against people and animals was one of four factors linked to persistent antisocial behavior over time. In a national sample, Vaughn et al. (2009) examined the lifetime prevalence of animal abuse and found significant associations with antisocial behaviors, as well as family history of antisocial behavior. Henry and Sanders (2007) found that both perpetrators and victims of bullying were more likely to abuse animals. Several studies suggest that recurrent animal abuse may serve as a better predictor than isolated acts of animal abuse (Hensley, Tallichet, & Dutkiewicz, 2009; Tallichet & Hensley, 2004).

1.4   Animal Abuse and Family Violence

Another strand of research indicates a strong association between animal abuse and family violence. The co-occurrence rate of physical child abuse and animal abuse is over 80 % (Deviney, Dickert, & Lockwood, 1983). Reviewing the research on the relationship between violence to children and violence to animals, Boat (1995) adds that there are many anecdotal reports linking animal abuse to the battering of women, sexual abuse of children, and acts of bestiality. There were similar findings for intimate partner violence. Ascione (2007) summarizes 12 interview studies of women seeking shelter in which up to 84 % reported that their partners had threatened, injured, or killed one or more family pets. In these studies, 29–76 % of children had been exposed to animal abuse, and up to 57 % of children had engaged in animal abuse themselves. DeGue and DiLillo (2009) interviewed college students, finding that 60 % of those who had been exposed to or engaged in animal abuse as children had also experienced child abuse or family violence. A large-scale study by Walton-Moss, Manganello, Frye, and Campbell (2005) found pet abuse to be one of the major risk factors for perpetrating intimate partner violence. Batterers who also abuse animals may also demonstrate more controlling behaviors and a wider range of abusive behaviors (Simmons & Lehmann, 2007).

The relationship between animal abuse and family violence is an important one, with implications for a variety of professional groups. However, children who engage in animal abuse do not necessarily come from violent families. The number of children who abuse animals is alarmingly high, as recent research discussed below has shown. Due to the prevalence of juvenile animal abuse and its developmental and clinical implications, all those who work with children need to be diligent about looking and listening for reports of animal abuse by children.

1.5   The Prevalence of Juvenile Animal Abuse

There are a number of well-designed studies that offer information on the prevalence of juvenile animal abuse. In general, the findings demonstrate that animal abuse in childhood is common. In the prevalence research, animal abuse was defined as deliberately hurting, torturing, or killing an animal in a cruel way.

Three studies of adult subjects, one of military personnel and the other two of college students, reported that 10–34.5 % of males admitted committing acts of animal abuse as children and 27–48.8 % had witnessed it (the lower rate came from the military sample) (Baker, Boat, Grinvalsky, & Geraciotti, 1998; Flynn, 1999; Miller & Knutson, 1997). All of these research subjects were functioning in society and, presumably, many did not come from violent families. Family violence is not the only factor associated with childhood animal abuse. Other studies on the incidence of juvenile animal abuse, which involved younger subjects, 2–18 years of age, indicated slightly different rates. Ascione (2001) reported on two studies with prevalence findings. The first, using the Achenbach-Conners-Quay Behavior Checklist, surveyed the parents of 2,600 boys and girls referred to mental health clinics for behavioral problems, who were compared to a control group of 2,600 boys and girls of the same age (ages 4–16). In the non-referred sample, the rate for animal abuse ranged from 0 to 6 % for girls and 4 to 13 % for boys; this contrasted to the referred sample in which the range was 7–17 % for girls and 18–34 % for boys. In addition to this survey, data for children ages 2–18 from the manuals of the Child Behavior Checklist indicated the following: The range of referred boys who reported incidents of animal abuse was 16–40 % and 9–31 % for referred girls. This compares to an animal abuse rate that ranged from 3 to 15 % for non-referred boys and 1 to 9 % for non-referred girls. Unlike the studies of the college and military samples referred to earlier, there was no definition of animal abuse and the time frame was limited to the past 2–6 months. Additionally, as Ascione noted (2001), caretakers typically underreport children's cruelty to animals.

What attitudes are associated with committing animal abuse? In one of the samples of college subjects, the researcher also asked, "Is it OK to slap your wife?" or "Is it OK to spank your children?" Individuals who had engaged in animal abuse as children were more likely to say "yes" to both of these questions (Flynn, 1999).

Children who abuse animals may not become serial killers, school shooters, batterers, or adult criminals—but they do become conditioned to accept and engage in interpersonal violence as adults. Even children who only witness animal abuse by family members or peers more often perpetrate animal abuse than non-witnesses (Baldry, 2003; Henry, 2004; Thomas & Gullone, 2006). They also report long-standing, recurring negative symptoms. Flynn's study of college students found that eight out of nine who had witnessed animal abuse as children reported being bothered "some" or "a lot" when the cruelty occurred and 73 % indicated it still bothered them (2000, p. 90). Assessing whether children have witnessed animal abuse is an important part of any evaluation of children and is discussed in the Treatment section.

1.6   Changing Attitudes Toward Animal Abuse

The pervasiveness of childhood animal abuse suggests, perhaps, that there has been a lack of recognition by some that animal abuse is another form of violence and that it requires a strong and immediate response by law enforcement, educators, parents, and mental health professionals. But that is changing. A growing awareness of the seriousness of animal abuse and its link to human violence has led to changes in animal abuse laws. Before 1990, only seven states had felony provisions in their animal cruelty laws; currently, 47 states and the District of Columbia have felony-level statutes. In about 30 states, the District of Columbia legislation allows, and in some instances mandates, the judge to include treatment as part of the sentence. In California, anyone convicted of animal abuse is required to receive treatment. In Illinois, Maine, Nevada, Texas, and Utah, treatment is mandated for juveniles, and in Iowa and New Mexico, the court "shall order" counseling for youth.

Other policies that recognize animal abuse are the development of "safe havens" that provide housing and care for companion animals of the human victims of domestic violence and court-ordered protective orders that include companion animals who were or are at risk of becoming co-victims of domestic violence.

As summarized above, research studies demonstrate various ways in which animal abuse is linked to violence against humans and other criminal and socially deviant behavior, as well as long-term mental health consequences that result from witnessing it. One important way to address the problem of youth violence is therefore to respond to animal abuse by reporting, investigating, prosecuting, and treating those who have perpetrated or witnessed abuse.

Throughout the years, clinicians who have treated children have encountered children who abuse animals. There is little research to ascertain how many clinicians evaluated their child clients to determine if they abused animals or witnessed abuse. However, a recent study of social workers found that one-third are including questions about companion and other animals in their intake assessments, and, although very few have had any special training, a bit less than 25 % are including companion and other animals in their intervention practice (Risley-Curtiss, 2010).

Very few clinicians treat the animal abuse as a central behavior to be addressed, just as they would directly address other forms of aggressiveness or sexual acting out or any other serious behavioral problem. Until recently, most clinicians viewed animal abuse more as a symptom than a behavior to be treated directly. Cruelty to animals was not added to the list of indicators for a diagnosis of conduct disorder in the Diagnostic and Statistical Manual of Mental Disorders until 1987 (DSM-IIIR). It has only been in the last decade that the research findings on the link between animal abuse and human violence have begun to be widely disseminated to professional audiences and the public.

Just as clinicians learned the importance of assessing and treating sexual abuse, substance disorders, and child abuse, now clinicians are much more prepared to understand the significance of animal abuse and to incorporate this knowledge into their practice. The purpose of *AniCare Child* is to provide clinicians with practical, clinically useful information about the assessment and treatment of children who have perpetrated or witnessed animal abuse.

Parents and others seek help for children who exhibit problems in behavior, social relationships, and other aspects of their lives, yet there is a marked scarcity of outcome research on therapy with children. For example, only 7.3 % of more than 3,000 studies looked into outcomes for children's therapy. A similar review corroborated these findings—only 6 % of an examined 15,000 studies focused on children's treatment outcomes (Christophersen & Mortweet, 2001).

Despite this lack of outcome data, there has been a movement over the last 30 years to support empirically researched treatments. The American Psychological Association Task Force on Empirically Supported Treatments recognized several procedures for the treatment of children they considered "well established" or "probably efficacious." Among these were cognitive problem-solving skills training and parent management training for oppositional and aggressive children (Christophersen & Mortweet 2001). Additionally, the Center for the Study and Prevention of Violence (CSPV) at the University of Colorado identified ten violence prevention programs that met a high scientific standard for program effectiveness. Other efforts also have focused on effective interventions for children (Kernberg & Chazan, 1991; Moeller, 2001).

AniCare Child draws upon this literature, as well as the experience of expert clinicians, to develop the interventions presented in the following sections. A direct evaluation of the effectiveness of *AniCare Child* is in process involving a mixed methodology of a case study and before/after/follow-up measures of several relevant variables ñ attitudes toward violence, attitudes toward animals, and empathy. In addition to this direct evaluation, the approach has indirect validation through its use of validated interventions for antisocial behaviors, particularly the work of Kazdin and his associates at Yale (Kazdin, Bass, Siegel, & Thomas, 1989; Kazdin, Siegel, & Bass, 1992; Kazdin & Weisz, 1998).

Theory

From our experience conducting AniCare workshops, it is clear that most therapists consider themselves either eclectic, employing a mix of theoretical approaches, or atheoretical, pragmatically providing whatever intervention they feel their client needs.

In this spirit, the handbook is organized by client function or skill, although several theories do inform the selection of interventions. Here we describe these, beginning with attachment theory, as we feel it is most helpful in formulating cases involving animal abuse. In turn, the other theories discussed are cognitive behavioral therapy (CBT), particularly personal narrative work, and psychodynamic theory.

2.1 Attachment Theory

Attachment theory was originated by John Bowlby to explain an individual's tendency to form strong emotional bonds to a particular individual, seen as providing protection, comfort, and security (Bowlby 1973, 1984, 1988). Bowlby proposed that infants are biologically predisposed to maintain closeness to an attachment figure by showing attachment behaviors that are designed to foster closeness, such as crying, clinging, or reaching out. Complementarily, caretakers are biologically disposed to respond to those infant signals with nurturance and caretaking.

Relationship experiences with caretakers result in relatively stable internal working models—a set of expectations that reflect the extent to which individuals believe themselves worthy of love and attention from others and the extent to which they believe that others will be available and supportive. These internal representations are incorporated into the developing personality structure and guide the formation of interpersonal relationships generally.

The premise that internal working models are continually shaped and reformulated by relationships throughout the life span offers promise for changing insecure models through therapy. A child who has negative models of self and other might experience a very different relationship with a therapist who offers a safe haven and

K. Shapiro et al., *The Assessment and Treatment of Children Who Abuse Animals*,
DOI 10.1007/978-3-319-01089-2_2, © Springer International Publishing Switzerland 2014

secure base. Ultimately, the child might be able to construct new models to guide future relationships outside of therapy.

From this base, therapists can weave a number of attachment-related questions into their assessment and treatment. For example: Are clients capable of forming an attachment relationship? How does the client's relationship with a companion animal relate to his or her human attachment relationships? Might a companion animal provide a secure base for an individual who has inadequate parental support? Are caretaking behaviors evident toward companion animals or the animal the client has abused?

The following schematic illustrates how attachment theory forms the basis of the AniCare approach. At the bottom of the scheme is Attachment—the development of secure or insecure attachments and their internalization to form internal working models. At the second level, and dependent on the quality of attachment, is sensitivity to one's own and others' feelings and capacity for empathy. Taken together, these are the basis for the level of Emotional Intelligence. At the third level, and dependent on the first two levels, are Self-Management Skills. At the fourth level, and feeding into all of the above, is Influence of Family and Subculture.

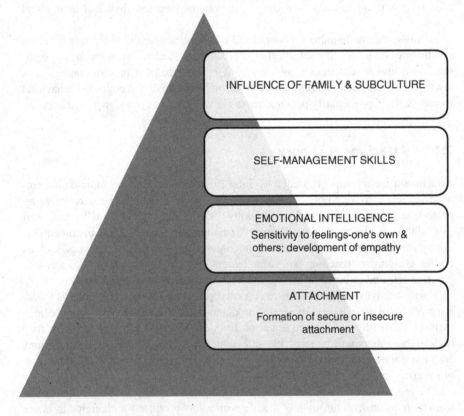

INFLUENCE OF FAMILY & SUBCULTURE

SELF-MANAGEMENT SKILLS

EMOTIONAL INTELLIGENCE
Sensitivity to feelings-one's own & others; development of empathy

ATTACHMENT
Formation of secure or insecure attachment

2.2   Cognitive Behavioral Therapy and Trauma-Informed Narrative

Cognitive behavioral therapy (CBT) is a familiar and highly validated set of inter-ventions based on the view that cognitions, themselves consisting of complexly related thoughts and feelings, interact in complex ways with behaviors. A change in either a cognition or a behavior can produce a change in the other. Therapists using this approach typically teach concrete skills to change or reframe thinking (such as self-management techniques) and behavioral strategies (such as problem-solving techniques).

A recent development in CBT featured in AniCare Child, trauma-focused cogni-tive behavior therapy is a versatile evidence-based best practice approach that may have benefits in the treatment of children with animal abuse histories. TF-CBT helps children with past or co-occurring trauma and externalized behavior, such as perpetrating animal abuse, to rebuild a narrative that is more integrative and health-ful (Cohen, Mannarino, & Deblinger, 2006).

Every child has a story to tell, and some of a child's earliest memories can become building blocks in the development of positive and secure attachments to both humans and animals. Many children who have abused animals have experienced earlier traumatic events that threatened their basic sense of security and safety. As a result, these children struggle with maturational challenges in the areas of attachment and affect regulation that impact their human-animal connections. The focus of narrative work with children with a history of trauma is to assist them in gaining a sense of "authorship" over their own lives and in making connections with both their positive and negative interactions with animals.

2.3   Psychodynamic Theory

A later development of psychoanalysis, psychodynamic theory emphasizes the sig-nificance of interpersonal relationships, particularly early and conflicted relation-ships, in the formation of a child's personality. Through analysis of patterns of past and present interpersonal relationships, including the relation to the therapist, the therapy helps the child to recognize needs and feelings and to find more prosocial ways of meeting and expressing them. The use of puppet role-play and projective techniques in the handbook, such as the Animals-at-Risk Thematic Apperception Test, generates material that is grist for psychodynamic analysis, including attach-ment issues.

Assessment

Regardless of the presenting problem, all children entering counseling should be assessed to determine if they have committed or witnessed acts of animal abuse. Children will be referred to counseling from a variety of sources: schools, parents, primary care physicians, district attorneys, probation departments, children's protection services, domestic violence agencies, church-based groups, and other community agencies. No matter what the referral source and presenting problem are, it is critical to determine if animal abuse is involved; however minor or major its role, it is imperative that addressing it be included in the treatment plan.

AniCare Child includes two assessment instruments devoted to the behavior of animal abuse: the Animal-Related Experiences Inventory and Factors to Consider in the Assessment of Animal Abuse (Factors to Consider). The first is a general screening device that should be used with all children referred for assessment with any presenting problem. The second is more fine-grained and is used to understand the nature and extent of the animal abuse.

Of course, these two devoted instruments will typically be used in conjunction with others that the therapist employs in his or her general practice. Taken together, the therapist can determine the centrality of animal abuse in a particular case. As we will discuss below in the Treatment section, for some children, the AniCare approach will be the primary treatment of choice, while for others it will augment other major interventions. For example, when working with a child with a major affective disorder or personality disorder, the therapist can select interventions from *AniCare Child* as needed in the context of the larger treatment program. On the other hand, when working with a child whose animal abuse is largely reactive to familial or other environmental situations, *AniCare Child* would be the primary treatment, perhaps supplemented by family meetings.

With these considerations in mind, we provide the following four-step approach to the assessment of juvenile animal abuse:

1. Ask about the child's relationship with animals
2. Obtain data from multiple sources

K. Shapiro et al., *The Assessment and Treatment of Children Who Abuse Animals,*   11
DOI 10.1007/978-3-319-01089-2_3, © Springer International Publishing Switzerland 2014

3. If the child perpetrated animal abuse, conduct a comprehensive assessment of the extent, nature, and motivation for animal abuse
4. If the child witnessed animal abuse, assess the effects

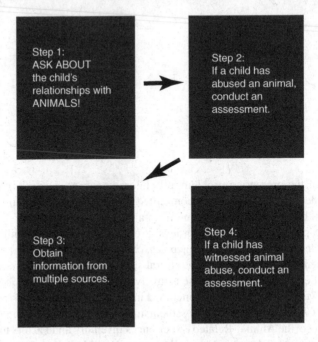

3.1   Steps in the Assessment of Animal Abuse

3.1.1   Step 1: ASK ABOUT the Child's Relationships with ANIMALS!

Assessment of ALL children, regardless of the presenting problem and referring agent, should include inquiry into their relationship with animals. Has the child perpetrated or witnessed abuse? Have animals been used by an adult or older child to coerce or control the child? Does the child fear animals? Has the child suffered the loss of an animal? Has an animal been an important attachment figure in his or her development?

To approach these issues, we recommend the "Animal-Related Experiences" Inventory (Inventory; Appendix A, pp. 81–85).

In addition to the questions on the inventory, to gain insight into what role pets play within the family, the clinician also can ask the child the following questions:
• What happens when your pet or companion animal misbehaves? Who disciplines him or her? How? What happens then?
• Have you ever been punished for something your pet did, like getting into the trash? Or has your pet ever been punished for something you did, like not doing the dishes when you were told to?

The clinician can closely adhere to the questions in the inventory or can embed them in a more free-flowing interview. What is important is to ask specific questions about a child's relationship with animals and to do so with the same inquisitive directness as one would ask about family relationships, sexual matters, possible abuse, suicidal feelings, or fantasy life.

> "Assessment interview with Michael" (Demonstration DVD, Assessment submenu) illustrates the use of the "Animal-Related Experiences" Inventory (Appendix A, pp. 81–85) in the context of an initial session.

Children frequently respond favorably when asked questions about animals in their lives; they often feel freer to talk about animals than themselves and subsequently can show more willingness to explore their thoughts and feelings.

Animals as a focus of the intervention also can be a potent tool for the therapist. Barbara Boat described how, in working with an adolescent girl from a severely abusive family, the girl's concern for her animals' welfare became a focus of the intervention. The girl's dog and two cats were an important source of support and could not accompany her to foster care. The therapist explored her feelings about the animals and helped her devise ways in which she might protect them. For example, the local SPCA was called in, determined that the dog was neglected, and relocated the dog to a safer environment. Safeguarding her animals gave them something the girl had been denied—protection and care. This option not only reduced the girl's anxiety but also empowered her to be effective and preserved her capacity for attachment.

Another clinician, Richard Ruth, reported that when working with children whose parents are able to function in their parental role, he speaks to the parents about the need for them to ensure the well-being of animals in the home. He explains that by protecting the animal, the parents are assuming an important parental function that aids in the child's recovery—establishing safety, protecting the dependent, and learning to care. In several situations in which there was an episode of animal abuse in the household, the parents and child came together to think about and care for the affected animal.

Some clinicians expand the inquiry into the child's relationships with animals by observing the child interact with animals—either their own pets or a pet therapy animal.

If there are companion animals at home, the clinician can ask the children to bring them into a session. She or he then observes how the child interacts with the animal and, just as importantly, how the animal reacts to the child. After a few sessions, one therapist instructed Kenneth, a 9-year-old referred to her for using a pit bull to kill a neighbor's rabbit, to bring his family pets, a dog and a cat, to a session.

Before Kenneth brought his pets into a session, the therapist had learned from his mother that Kenneth had caused minor injuries to them, cutting the whiskers off of the cat's face and using tweezers to pull out the dog's whiskers. Kenneth also had maimed a pet hamster by cutting her toes off and seriously injured a classroom turtle under his care for the weekend by pinching his toes off.

When the family's pets entered the session, the cat immediately hid underneath the desk (not unusual behavior for a cat). The dog appeared leery of Kenneth, yet friendly with the therapist, staying close to her. The young man exhibited little interest in the animals. Occasionally he would order his dog to "Sit down!" or "Come over here!" Other than issuing occasional commands, he mostly ignored them. When the therapist asked him their names, he responded with a one-word response. When she inquired further, "What are they like?" or "How would you describe their personalities?" he shrugged his shoulders and seemed uninterested in talking about them.

Further attempts to question Kenneth about his relationship with the family pets were not successful. The therapist used the information she gleaned from this session, along with other clinical impressions, to conjecture that Kenneth had serious difficulty forming attachments and a reduced capacity for empathy.

Therapists who work with animal therapists, such as Susan Krinsk, whose co-therapist is a 160-pound bull mastiff named Taz, routinely gain information by observing the child's reaction to him. For example, she learns a great deal about a child's ability to form attachments, observe boundaries, understand another's perspective, and postpone his or her own immediate needs. She then uses the child's interactions with Taz to help the child develop skills in necessary areas.

In summary, the basic principle for making an assessment is Ask! If a child has been referred for animal abuse or if perpetration or witnessing of animal abuse is detected in the assessment, the next step is to make a thorough evaluation of the various factors that may be contributing to this behavior.

3.1.2   Step 2: If a Child Has Abused an Animal, Conduct an Assessment

First, what is animal abuse? A general definition by Ascione offers a useful framework: "Socially unacceptable non-accidental behavior that causes unnecessary pain, suffering, distress, or death" (Ascione & Shapiro, 2009). The term "socially unacceptable" excludes as animal abuse many institutionalized forms of treatment of animals that are the object of concern in the contemporary animal protection movement. However, it also assures that the definition is historically evolving and culturally contingent. Note that most of the empirical literature on the relationship between animal abuse and other forms of violence is based on the mistreatment of companion animals in the home. Also, note that the term "non-accidental" includes as abuse neglectful behavior, the most common form of animal abuse.

This general definition needs elaboration to be useful to the clinician in determining whether animal abuse has occurred, the degree of seriousness of the abuse, and the risk of further aggression toward animals and people.

• Andy, a 3-year-old boy in preschool, pulls on the classroom rabbit's ears.
• Alice is 18 years old. She ties her dog to his doghouse and frequently leaves him alone without appropriate shelter.
• Sam is walking down the street with his pit bull. When he sees another boy from his neighborhood with a dog, he challenges him to a dogfight. They take their dogs to a nearby alley, unleash them, and watch the dogs fight.

- Martin, an 11-year-old, hangs out with three other boys, two of whom are 12 years old and one who is his age. On the way home from school, one of the older boys dares Martin to grab a cat who is sunning herself on the steps of the animal's home. After Martin does this, the boys throw the cat in a bag and begin to throw the cat around like a ball. One of the boys, who has a bat, begins to hit the bagged animal like a baseball.
- George, a 13-year-old, entered a shelter with three other boys and bludgeoned 18 cats to death. George was perplexed by his arrest and his requirement to undergo counseling, stating "They were only cats!" His sentiment that "they were only cats" was shared by his friends and family.

The above examples give a sense of the range of possible animal mistreatment and suggest some of the factors that need to be considered.

3.1.3   Factors to Consider in the Assessment of Juvenile Animal Abuse

Within the context of a thorough psychosocial assessment of the child, there are a number of factors to consider in assessing a child who has mistreated an animal. Organized into categories of severity, culpability, psychodynamics and motivation, attitudes/beliefs, emotional intelligence, family history, and mitigating circumstances, the factors (p. 17) complement the Animal-Related Experiences Inventory by providing a framework for the assessment. They do not represent an exhaustive and mutually exclusive set of variables and are continually being updated to reflect advances in research and clinical experience. They address a number of important areas that deserve careful assessment and that are helpful in formulating interventions.

The assessment of animal abuse might identify factors in more than one category; the categories are not mutually exclusive. For example, the age or developmental level of the child, a factor in culpability, could overlap with the motivational factor of curiosity or experimentation. Additionally, factors within categories might be highly correlated. Narcissistic slights/rage and the motivation to alleviate feelings of powerlessness can co-occur with feelings of impotence in the category of psychodynamics/motivation. Some factors may appear in two categories—such as capacity for forming a secure attachment—which may be considered both a mitigating circumstance and an indication of emotional intelligence.

The categories of degree of severity and extent of culpability give an indication of the level of intervention that might be necessary. A young child who committed a solitary act of mishandling an animal—such as pulling the family cat's tail—that inflicted little or no injury, and who did not plan or clearly understand his actions, would require a very different level of intervention than an older adolescent who committed repeated acts of animal abuse against a number of species. In the first case, an intervention by parents that modeled responsible interactions with the pet and the need for them to be monitored might be sufficient. In the example of the adolescent, a more extensive intervention, including psychotherapy, would be strongly recommended.

The psychodynamics and motivation for the abuse will offer insight into the psychological makeup of the child, help the clinician understand the child's experience, and influence the type and timing of interventions. For example, the child's motivation could be more reactive—responding to a perceived environmental threat, such as fear of an animal or to peer pressure—than instrumental, using aggression for a particular purpose, such as coercion or enhancing one's own aggressiveness. Interventions for a reactive child might focus more on self-management skills—gaining impulse control, improving problem-solving skills, or providing safe and positive exposure to the feared animal. The child whose abuse tends to be more instrumental might require more of an emphasis on the development of emotional sensitivity and expressivity and empathy (Moéller, 2001). (See the empathy/self-management schema, p. 25.) Motivations that have a strong physiological component, such as mood enhancement or sexual arousal, might require yet another approach that addresses the biology of the motivation and an evaluation for medication may also be indicated.

Therapy, especially with children, could involve psycho-education; for example, humane education, cognitive reframing, and socio-emotional development. Assessing the child's attitudes and beliefs about animals can help the clinician understand what misconceptions might need to be addressed. For example, many children and adults might not be aware of the physical and psychological needs of an animal or, because of implicit acceptance of subcultural norms, may harbor prejudice against a particular species, such as cats. Clarifying and rectifying the child's attitudes and beliefs can help lay the foundation for therapeutic work on developing the child's emotional intelligence. For example, a child will need some basic information on an animal's physical and psychological needs in order to develop a capacity for empathy.

In the past 20 years, clinicians have learned to include direct questions about abuse and family discipline in their assessments. The known co-occurrence of animal abuse and family violence, as well as animal abuse and physical punishment of children, confirms the necessity of including questions about the treatment of animals in the household.

Assessing mitigating circumstances and assets adds important information and assists the clinician to determine the quality of the child's socio-emotional functioning, capacity for empathy, and moral development.

Finally, if the child presents a danger to a family pet, be sure that the parents separate the child from the pet, allowing only highly supervised, limited contact. Work out a safety plan for the animal with the parents. If there are no family pets, strongly urge the parents not to obtain any until the child can be trusted.

3.1.4   Step 3: Obtain Information from Multiple Sources

As much as possible, obtain data from multiple sources. Often children with behavioral problems require a multisystematic approach to treatment; therefore, it is useful to contact other involved individuals and agencies when making the assessment.

Factors to consider in the assessment of juvenile animal abuse[a]

Severity

Degree of injury (mild, moderate, severe)

Frequency and duration (how many times, over what span of time)

Number and kind of species, including level of sentience (degree to which an animal is capable of sensation or feeling)

Prolonged or immediate

Intimacy of infliction of injury—stabbed or shot at distance

Culpability

Age/developmental level: Were consequences understood?

Knowledge of what constitutes a criminal act? Awareness of extent of animal suffering?

Degree of planning

Obstacles that were overcome

Alone or in a group: if in group, leader or follower?

Coercion by a more dominant individual

Psychodynamics/motivation

Curiosity/experimentation

Reaction to fear of animal

To coerce or retaliate against a human

Reaction to personal experience of abuse/punishment (post-traumatic attempt for mastery/control; identification with the aggressor; displacement of aggression)

Peer pressure (culture of hypermasculinity)

Other antisocial behavior (aggression in family, with peers, or strangers; property crime; drug-related offenses)

Profit motive, commercial gain

Rehearsing or enhancing one's own aggressiveness

Hypersensitivity to real or perceived threats

Insensitive to or callous about or dissociated from suffering of the abused animal(s)

Target of abuse own companion animal

Target of abuse neighbor's or unknown animal

Abused animal primary target

Abused animal substitute or displaced target

Hypersensitivity to rejection

Narcissistic slights/rage

Alleviate feelings of powerlessness, loneliness, or alienation

Mood enhancement (relief from boredom or depression)

Pleasure from inflicting suffering (sadism)

Sexual assault of an animal and/or sexual arousal resulted from abuse

Documented abuse with video or photograph and/or returned to scene to relive

Ritualistic features

Attitudes/beliefs

Unaware of the physical and psychological needs of animals and how they differ by species

Believes that animals exist for instrumental purposes only

Has given little or no thought to the roles and positions of animals in human society

Prejudice against a particular species (e.g., cats)

Cruelty as a way to control and "discipline" an animal

Cultural practice or acceptance

Emotional intelligence

Capable of identifying and expressing feelings

Capable of empathy

Capable of reciprocal relationship

Understanding of relationships—need to reciprocate, accommodate

Capable of forming secure attachments

Resilience and readiness to change

Family history

Domestic violence

Child abuse

Physical or emotional neglect

Animal abuse

Harsh and inconsistent discipline

Spanking and other physical punishment

Mitigating circumstances

Accepts responsibility

Expresses feelings of remorse, shame, or guilt

Seeks to make restitution

Assists law enforcement

Capable of forming bond with an animal

[a]These factors were derived from a variety of sources, including Arluke (1997); Ascione (2001); Ascione, Thompson, and Black (1997); Bickerstaff (2003); Boat (1999); Gupta (2008); Jory and Randour (1999); Kellert and Felthous (1985); Lewchanin and Zimmerman (2000); and Lockwood (1998)

AniCare Child recommends that clinicians seek permission to obtain information from, or share information with, the following parties:

- Parents
- Teachers
- Guidance counselors
- Medical and court records
- Psychological evaluations
- Pediatricians
- Other family members
- Previous school
- Principal
- Social worker
- Neighborhood friends
- Veterinarian

3.1.5   Involving Parents in the Assessment

Research clearly demonstrates that parent and family characteristics are essentially related to the development of antisocial behavior in children. Parental stress, psychopathology, social isolation, poor parental relations, child-rearing practices, depression, and substance abuse contribute to aggressive behavior in children (Kazdin, 1995; Robins, 1991; Rutter & Giller, 1983).

In the parent assessment, the clinician seeks information about the child, the parents' psychology as individuals and as parents, and the family system, including the role of any companion animals in the family.

The inventory can be used with the parents to gain information about the child's relationship with animals. As with the child interview, when assessing parents, *AniCare Child* suggests adding the following questions to those found in the inventory:

- What happens when the family pet misbehaves? Who disciplines him or her? How? What happens then?
- Do you ever punish your child for something the pet did?
- How many pets have you had in your family? What happened to them?
- Who do you think should have the responsibility for the pet in your family?

Clinicians who work with children and their families often use a variety of other assessment tools—standardized tests, checklists, inventories, and questionnaires. These should be used as needed to complement the two assessment instruments in *AniCare Child* and to gain information about the child from the parent, as well as from teachers and the child directly.

There also are a number of instruments that are easily administered and that provide useful information about the parents. A psychosocial evaluation for use with parents is Appendix B, pp. 76–82.

3.1.6 Step 4: If a Child Has Witnessed Animal Abuse, Conduct an Assessment

As noted earlier, witnessing animal abuse is a common experience in childhood and one that has significant consequences for the witness. Many children report negative emotions suggestive of post-traumatic stress. However, witnesses also more often subsequently perpetrate abuse than non-witnesses. Both gender and age are relevant variables: Girls more often become more sensitive while men more often become more callous toward animals following witnessing. The age-related finding is that children who observe animal abuse before the age of 12 are more likely to become perpetrators than those who observe after age 12 (Henry, 2004).

Witnessing itself can blur with perpetration as when an individual is part of a group of perpetrators but does not himself/herself actively contribute to the abuse. The focus of the literature on witnessing is on cases where the individual is not a member of a group that abuses, but rather is forced to observe, or is intentionally or incidentally exposed. Children can witness animal abuse but not be directly involved in the action or may be a part of a group in which some members actively engage in cruelty toward an animal. For example, one study found that over 50 % of children who commit animal abuse do so in a group of two or more (Luke, Arluke, & Levin, 1997). Additionally, some children witness animal abuse in their homes that is often committed by a parent or older sibling. In cases of family violence, animal abuse often is used to punish or intimidate other family members (Flynn, 2000).

> "Empathy Skills" (Demonstration DVD, submenu Treatment), with Joel, illustrates a case (Joel) of possible "forced to observe" or at least reluctant to observe; Appendix E (pp. 107–115), Jeremy, illustrates case of "incidentally exposed."

If the child witnessed animal abuse, obtain the details of the abuse. Ascertain the following:
- The relationship of the child to the abuser; if he or she was a family member, do a thorough assessment of other abuse that could be occurring in the family and take appropriate action
- The relationship of the child to the animal
- The type and severity of the abuse and who was involved
- How many times it occurred
- The type of victim(s), and the victim(s) response, as well as the response of the perpetrators and other witnesses
- What, if anything, bothered the child the most about what happened

Determine the child's role in witnessing animal abuse. Was she or he passive, encouraging, or coerced (real or perceived)?

Ask the child, "How do you feel about being involved in what happened?"

Assess the child's immediate and long-term response to being a witness.

Ask the child about mental, physical, emotional, or behavioral reactions and symptoms immediately following the incident and what he or she is experiencing now.

Determine if the child is suffering from any symptoms of post-traumatic stress disorder (PTSD).

Does the child exhibit the following:
- Anxiety
- Nightmares or frightening dreams
- Difficulty sleeping or eating
- Problems concentrating
- Repetitive play with themes or aspects of the trauma
- Disorganized or agitated behavior

Does the child feel the following:
- Shame
- Guilt
- Remorse

Does the child experience the following:
- Numbing or feelings of detachment
- A restricted range of affect

Is the child fearful of reprisal?

Did the child report the abuse to anyone?

What was the response of the person to whom the child reported the abuse?

3.1.7 Conclusion

The central principle of any assessment is to ask about animals in a child's life—past or present. If abuse is discovered, conduct a thorough assessment of the abuse to determine culpability, motivation, attitudes and beliefs, emotional intelligence, family history, and mitigating circumstances. In addition to the clinical interview of the child, include data from multiple sources, especially parents. Administer supplemental instruments as needed to assess possible substance abuse, personality disorder, or other psychopathology. Finally, in any assessment, ask about a child's exposure to animal abuse as a witness.

Use the several cases described and analyzed in the text of the handbook to practice assessment, including case formulation, diagnosis (see immediately below), and recommendations for intervention. Supplemental case material is provided in Appendix E (pp. 107–115) and in the Demonstration DVD (see both Assessment and Treatment submenus).

One general purpose of an assessment is to provide a psychological (and sociocultural) portrait of a juvenile who has abused animals. The portrait can be framed in experiential terms (the "world-as-lived" by a person who abuses animals) or clinical terms ("psychopathology," "personality," "theory") or more strictly in treatment planning and objectives terms.

If animal abuse or the witnessing of animal abuse is present, some form of intervention is necessary. As in any assessment context, the evaluator should consider recommendation of the full spectrum of possible interventions. Obviously, not all children who abuse animals are appropriate referrals for *AniCare Child*. Levels of intervention include, from minimal to most intense and extensive, education, parent guidance, psycho-education, diversion program, counseling, medication, and part-time or full-time residential placement. An example of a psycho-education intervention is Project Second Chance (PSC), which provides juveniles in residence for antisocial behavior with a companion animal from a shelter. Each youth is supervised in training a dog and taught responsible caretaking along with such skills as empathy and accountability. Children and Animals Together (CAT), an example of a diversion program, includes an assessment and a 14-week intervention group held at a local animal shelter. CAT can be used in conjunction with individual counseling or other interventions. Both PSC and CAT adapt techniques from *AniCare Child*. Green Chimneys is a residential treatment that provides children with major emotional and behavioral problems the resocialization opportunities offered by living on a working farm (see case of Calvin, pp. 44–47).

In addition to making a detailed assessment of the extent, nature, and motivation for animal abuse and, if witnessed, the emotional effects of observing it, also assess the child for a possible clinical diagnosis. Providing a diagnosis can help the therapist determine how AniCare should be used in a given case. Is it the treatment of choice, perhaps supplemented by other interventions, or is it itself a supplementary part of a broader treatment approach?

In our discussion of diagnostic categories, we rely on the *Diagnostic and Statistical Manual of Mental Disorders*, Fourth Edition (DSM-IV 1994).

3.2 Diagnostic Categories Associated with Children Who Commit Animal Abuse

3.2.1 Attention-Deficit and Disruptive Behavior Disorders

Researchers agree that aggression manifested early in life tends to be fairly stable and is the single best predictor of later criminal behavior (Cavell, 2000; Moeller, 2001). Developmental theorists posit two developmental pathways to conduct disorder (CD)—an early starter and later onset model (Kazdin, 1985; Loeber, 1991; Moffitt, 1993; Patterson, DeBaryshe, & Ramsey, 1989). Early-onset conduct disorder has a much worse prognosis than conduct disorder that begins in adolescence and accounts for a disproportionate number of delinquent acts in adolescence. In the early starter model, aggressive behavior emerges with oppositional defiant disorder (ODD) in the early preschool years, progresses to aggressive and nonaggressive (e.g., lying and stealing) behaviors during middle childhood, and then develops into the most serious behaviors in adolescence of interpersonal violence and property crimes (Lahey, Loeber, Quay, Frick, & Grimm, 1992).

Antisocial behavior appears to remain stable over the course of development, forecasts major dysfunction in adulthood, and is intergenerational in nature (Kazdin, Bass, Siegel, & Thomas, 1989). As many as 50 % of children diagnosed with conduct disorder show problems in adolescence and adulthood. These children also exhibit other problem behaviors in adulthood, including psychological disorders, substance abuse, poor occupational adjustment, lower education attainment, marital problems, poor interpersonal relationships, and problems with physical health (Loeber, 1990).

Experts agree that "the continuity of CD demonstrates the importance of programs that focus on prevention and early treatment of conduct problems" (Christophersen & Mortweet, 2001). Theorists convinced of the early-onset model suggest that the most strategic point for intervention in the child's development is in the preschool and early elementary school from 4 to 7 years of age. As aggressive children get older, they are increasingly less responsive to therapeutic interventions (Kazdin, 1995; Loeber, 1990). Again, since animal abuse often appears at an early age, identification and treatment provides for the possibility of earlier and more successful interventions.

It also should be noted that children demonstrating antisocial behavior and their families frequently drop out of treatment. For example, in one clinical study, 22 % of the cases dropped out of treatment (Kazdin, Siegel, & Bass 1992); in general, attrition in child therapy studies ranged from 45 to 65 % (Pekarik & Stephenson, 1988). In addition, various studies have determined that children who exhibit disruptive and aggressive behavior make up nearly 50 % of all child referrals for psychological services (Christophersen & Mortweet, 2001; McMahon & Forehand, 1984).

In general, the disruptive behavior diagnoses of CD, ODD, and attention-deficit/ hyperactivity disorder (ADHD) often coexist. Since animal abuse is one of the indicators for a diagnosis of CD and may be implicated in other behavior disorders, it is especially important to assess for animal abuse when evaluating children with behavioral disorders. It's critical to assess the severity of CD, as well as its presence, since the severity of aggressive behavior has predictive value: Higher levels of aggressiveness are predictive of criminal offenses in adulthood (Vitiello & Jensen, 1995). The severity of animal abuse, as well as the child's culpability and motivation, is an important factor in determining the degree of conduct disorder, whether mild, moderate, or severe. Other researchers distinguish between whether or not the aggression is reactive (a defensive reaction to a perceived threat, usually accompanied by displays of anger) or proactive (acts designed to achieve an instrumental goal, to possess an object, or to dominate another) (Dodge & Coie, 1987; Dodge & Crick, 1990). Many aggressive children display both types of aggression, but with some, very specific and directed interventions may be warranted. For example, treatments that concentrate on teaching self-management skills—self-control, self-monitoring, and problem-solving—may be more effective with the reactive aggressive child than the proactive one (Cavell, 2000).

In addition, the clinician should carefully conduct a differential diagnosis of CD, ODD, and ADHD. A diagnosis of disruptive behavior not otherwise specified also may be appropriate in some cases. Detailed comparisons of children with ODD and conduct disorder determined that most of the children who were diagnosed with conduct disorder also met diagnostic criteria for ODD; in one study it was reported that as many as 90 % of children with early-onset CD met the criteria for ODD (Vitiello & Jensen, 1995). Some have concluded that ODD is a more moderate variant of conduct disorder (Schachar & Wachsmuth, 1990). Most cases of CD have an onset at age 9, often preceded by ODD, which appears earlier, at approximately 6.5 years (Frick et al., 1993). The average age for onset of animal abuse also is 6.5, which suggests that earlier interventions for CD can be made if clinicians also assess and treat animal abuse in children.

Possible diagnoses should not be limited to those discussed above but, depending on the information obtained during the assessment, should include other possibilities such as anxiety disorders, including post-traumatic stress disorder, adjustment disorder, and mood disorders, as well as the various personality disorders, pervasive developmental disorders, mental retardation, and traumatic brain injury.

3.2.2 Attachment Difficulties

Although many children who engage in juvenile animal abuse will meet the criteria for ODD or CD, not all will. Clinicians also may want to consider difficulties with attachment, which may be associated with animal abuse.

3.2.3 Attachment Issues

Attachment issues are not currently codified in a discrete disorder in official diagnostic manuals. DSM-IV, which specifies the diagnostic criteria for reactive attachment disorder of infancy or early childhood, notes that the disorder appears to be uncommon (American Psychiatric Association, 1994). However, *AniCare Child* suggests that assessment of the child's capacity for attachment is critical to understanding and developing a treatment plan. For example, if a the clinician determines that a child has a diminished capacity to form secure attachments, she or he might pay particular attention to the development of a therapeutic relationship, with special sensitivity to missed sessions, time between sessions, and losses. When conferring with parents, the clinician might advise interventions designed to foster attachment—physical closeness and touching when engaged in positive interactions with the child. A finding that the child may exhibit attachment difficulties does not preclude a diagnosis of ODD or CD.

Another reason to consider the quality of a child's attachment is that underlying the *AniCare Child* dual focus on self-management and empathy development is a concern about moral development. Because there are research findings that link the capacity to attach to moral development (Moeller, 2001), *AniCare Child* finds utility in the exploration of the complex issues associated with attachment.

Finally, many clinicians believe that the capacity to attach provides an important prognostic tool for the course and success of treatment. Without a capacity for attachment or the capacity to learn to attach, the vital connection between therapist and client, so integral to the success of many treatments, may be in question. At the same time, it is important to recognize that there are many levels of connection between therapists and children, that therapeutic approaches can vary for different children, and that even small improvements in attachment can indicate progress or success.

Treatment

Animal abuse is similar to treatments for fire-setting, sexual misconduct, and substance abuse, in that the therapist will directly address the client's behavior—in this case cruelty to animals—in an explicit and direct way. When behaviors are aggressive, violent, antisocial, and dangerous to people and animals, an active therapeutic stance is recommended. In these cases, the therapist explicitly addresses the maladaptive behaviors and works with the client to replace these behaviors with more adaptive responses.

As discussed in Chap. 3, the interventions in *AniCare Child* can be the primary vehicle of treatment, or they can provide supplemental interventions in a treatment program with a broader focus, such as major affective disorder, a personality disorder, or developmental delay. That treatment may not be in an individual-based setting; it could be part of a family-based counseling intervention or a residential treatment program.

The treatment section of the handbook is organized under four components: connection (Sect. 4.1, pp. 26–33), empathy (Sect. 4.2, pp. 33–55; subdivided into identification/expression of feelings and empathy development), self-management (Sect. 4.3, pp. 55–89), and working with parents (Sect. 4.2, pp. 89–100). Although we present the four components in the suggested order of their use, it should be clear that AniCare is an approach, not a manual. The therapist must continually exercise his or her judgment about the order both across and within each component. Some examples:

1. An effective intervention is sometimes a necessary precondition for establishing the client's confidence in and connection to the therapist.
2. A client might be more oriented to the feelings of others (empathy) than to his or her own feelings.
3. A level of self-management can be a precondition for the client to have access to feelings of self and others.

Treatment of childhood animal abuse will resemble many other treatments for children, and therefore, the basic theoretical and clinical models of diagnosis and interventions will also apply to children who abuse animals. However, one distinguishing feature of a treatment that focuses on animal abuse, whether it is central to the treatment or one component of it, can be identified.

K. Shapiro et al., *The Assessment and Treatment of Children Who Abuse Animals*,   25
DOI 10.1007/978-3-319-01089-2_4, © Springer International Publishing Switzerland 2014

Animals and the child's relationship with them, attitudes toward them, beliefs about them, and learned behavior around them all will be a central feature in the treatment. In the course of the therapy, much discussion typically will involve animals. In addition, the therapist will introduce virtual or symbolic animals through exercises and projective instruments, including the use of puppets, play, and drawing. To teach certain skills, such as problem-solving, empathy, or self-management, exercises included throughout *AniCare Child* will emphasize situations with animals.

The use of actual animals can be a potent and effective intervention to teach boundaries, empathy, and foster attachment skills. However, since animal abuse is generally a psychologically laden issue for these clients, the use of animal-assisted therapy and activities must be undertaken with careful consideration of its likely benefits and possible risks. (See further discussion below under Sects. 4.1 and 4.2.1.7, pp. 26–33.) Whether through the indirect and/or direct use of animals, the primary goal of treatment is the elimination of animal abuse.

4.1   Connection

Connection refers to the important initial task of establishing a working therapeutic relationship. When there is a strong alliance, the client is more likely to engage in therapy, accept suggestions and interventions, explore thoughts and feelings, and experiment with new behaviors.

Developing the therapeutic alliance begins when the consulting room door opens and continues throughout treatment. It is not limited to particular techniques but infuses all interactions. This section presents four methods that clinicians can use to establish a nurturing therapeutic connection:

- Processing therapist reactions
- Joining the client
- Framing the therapy
- The indirect or direct use of animals

The methods presented in this section often overlap, the order of their use may be varied, and they are not meant to be exhaustive. Rather, these are suggested approaches for clinicians with varied backgrounds and for other professionals who will use the *AniCare Child* model.

4.1.1   Processing Therapist Reactions

Therapists who work with clients who harm others may find it difficult to hear about incidents in which violence was directed at an innocent being. On occasion, therapists will be faced with their own negative reactions—anger, grief, disgust, and outrage. When experiencing aversive reactions to the client, the therapist faces special challenges in making and maintaining the connection. While it is essential for a therapist to acknowledge these feelings, it is also crucial that therapists find ways to process them in order to remain available to help the client and to avoid demonizing or discounting the client in any way.

Countertransference, a concept from psychodynamic theory, refers to the feelings the therapist may have toward the client. Often these feelings are not in the therapist's full conscious awareness and may be a reflection of his or her own issues. This is a very real occupational hazard for therapists working with this population, since they often self-select because of their love of animals. These feelings can be subtle or quite strong.

One way in which therapists can process these feelings is by talking with a peer. Support groups or informal sessions with colleagues provide important support. In cases where the feelings are more persistent, or in which informal contact with colleagues has not resolved them, scheduled meetings with a supervisor or consultant are recommended.

Once worked through, the therapist may indirectly bring his or her feelings back into the therapy, assuming that the client arouses these feelings in others as well. For example, "It makes me feel uncomfortable when you say that. Do you think it may make other people around you uncomfortable? Were you aware of that? Can you become aware of it?"

Another strategy that therapists may use when confronted with their own reactions to the child's abusive behavior is to focus on an underlying feeling, such as shame, guilt, or anxiety, thereby bypassing the offending behavior. For example, Susan Krinsk often offers personal examples from her own life as a way to communicate that she understands and to build the therapeutic alliance. Noting that it is often very hard to acknowledge when you have done something bad because of feelings of shame and guilt, Krinsk might mention "I did things that were bad when I was younger and remembering those things is hard for me, too." She will share enough so the child knows that she can relate to them but clearly places limits on what she reveals. With younger children she offers more general references, saying "When I was young I didn't always see eye to eye with my parents," or, referring to the child's relationship to animals, Krinsk might observe, "Pets can be really frustrating sometimes. When I was a kid I used to want them to love me, whether they were in the mood or not. And I didn't like it when they wouldn't." She may supply somewhat more detail to teenaged clients, remarking, "When I was younger I got into trouble for not following directions and for being impatient. I thought I knew it all."

In rare instances, the therapist may need to recognize that he or she is not able to deal with a client and a referral is the better option.

4.1.2 Joining the Client

Using the child's own language indicates that the therapist understands the world from the child's perspective. If the child said he "wasted" an animal because his friends were "ragging on him," the therapist might use those exact words rather than resorting to more formal language, such as "injuring" the animal because friends were "taunting" you. Often the child's language will be more blunt than adult expressions and the therapist's use of the child's language can contribute to the child feeling understood. Additionally, the use of candid language or straight talk may help the child acknowledge the reality of the event and the seriousness of his or her actions.

One therapist first greeted Toby, a 13-year-old Caucasian boy sent to her for killing a squirrel, by saying, "So I get from the expression on your face that your week sucked." She also expressed understanding of Toby's desire to escape from adult authority. On one occasion she offered, "I bet you're glad it's snowing—school will be dismissed and you won't have to worry about any homework that isn't done. I used to look for the snow when I was a kid."

In addition to using the child's language, Deborah Matthews shows interest in the child's clothing, music, and other unique expressions of his or her personality or developing identity. She also will share some of her experiences as a child and adolescent to indicate that what the child is experiencing is not unusual.

Another way to join the child is to inquire into the child's reactions to the therapist. Deborah Matthews directly asks the child, "What is it like for you to talk to me?" Many children will have difficulty answering this and will require prompting and encouragement: "I can imagine that you have some feelings about being here and having me ask you questions about this. We are talking about something that got you into trouble." Or "What do you feel, or what goes through your mind, when I ask you questions about your situation?" This conveys to the child that the therapist is aware that his or her experience of therapy is a significant thing to talk about. It also prompts the child to pay attention to feelings, to identify them, and to use them for information. Finally, and most importantly, it focuses on the importance of the therapeutic relationship and the effect that the therapist and the client have on each other.

The therapists who provided case material for *AniCare Child* acknowledged that they used the child's language when they had general discussions with the child, even when that language might not be acceptable in other situations, such as in the classroom setting.

For example, depending on the context, they noted that they may pick up on a word or phrase the child uses, such as "So you think this is a real bummer" or "You looked pissed off to me" or "You said they screwed up, but it appears that you also screwed up pretty badly," and use that expression with the child. Susan Krinsk qualifies this adoption of the child's language by noting that at times she might caution the child about his or her language, urging the child to identify situations in which he or she may need to restrain him or herself.

At the same time that therapists are encouraged to use plain language when discussing abuse, clinicians need to adopt an attitude that implies neither judgment nor permissiveness. In cases of animal abuse, the subject of remorse and acceptance of responsibility will be a recurring one. Deborah Matthews describes a forthright approach to this topic. If the child is remorseful, she approaches the child very gently and quietly listens to his or her feelings of regret. However, if the child is not remorseful, she notes that. For example, she might say, "You know, coming to therapy means learning to accept responsibility for what you do."

One therapist explained that when she is working with clients who have been referred by the courts, she ends to be more direct than when she is treating patients who attend therapy voluntarily. With all clients, she begins by establishing basic limits and parameters of treatment. For example, at her initial meeting with Toby, she explained what he could and could not do in her office, saying, "You can talk about any thought or feeling—in fact, I hope you tell me everything that is on your mind. That is why you are here. We need to figure out what is going on inside you so we can find ways to help you deal better with your problems. However, you cannot do some things. You cannot try to threaten or intimidate, and you can't 'trash' my office." She also explains the limits of confidentiality, length of sessions, policy regarding missed sessions, and other issues related to the parameters of the therapy.

4.1.3 Framing the Therapy

Related to using a child's language and speaking frankly is knowing when to adopt a more formal or neutral demeanor. The connection with the child must be in the context of a relationship in which the therapist is able to work effectively with the client. The therapy should be structured so that the therapist can gain information, keep the client on task, and set limits so that the child feels protected and safe with firm boundaries. The therapist needs to balance the use of the child's language with the use of more formal, "adult" language, switching to this more serious demeanor in certain situations. When using a psycho-educational approach, therapists frequently use more formal, adult language so that when teaching sexual anatomy, functioning, and behaviors they use the correct terms and convey seriousness. Susan Krinsk notes that many of the children with whom she works lack basic information about sexual behavior, anatomy, and functioning, and she talks about these topics frankly and in detail. Sometimes, the children notice the sexual organs of Taz, her animal co-therapist, and ask questions; or she observes them looking at Taz and may say, "I noticed that you are looking at Taz's penis. Dogs don't wear clothes. Because they don't, we can notice their private parts and that may make us curious." From that discussion, she talks about private parts, the importance of respecting one's own and other's private parts, and taking responsibility for how we treat others. At the beginning of treatment, it is appropriate for clinicians to advise parents that they will be talking to their child frankly about sexual matters, such as masturbation, pregnancy, and sexual urges, and to secure parental permission to do so.

When setting boundaries or discussing legal matters, such as a court order, therapists typically use an earnest tone. The therapist also might use a more serious tone when engaged in a "reality check." The therapist who was treating Toby (sent to her for cruelly killing a squirrel) recollected that he mentioned that he wanted to get a pet squirrel.

Interpreting this as a test of the boundaries that had been established by the therapy, she replied, "That's not going to happen. Why do you think?" Toby claimed he couldn't understand why he couldn't have a squirrel. The therapist reminded him that his past contact with a squirrel had cast doubt on his behavior toward animals, that the courts were overseeing his behavior, and that no responsible adult would sanction his contact with a squirrel at this point. When talking to Toby, she adopted a serious tone to convey the shift from exploration to limit-setting.

4.1.4 Animal-Assisted Therapy

Animal-assisted activity (AAA) is a growing field that takes many forms—institutionally based programs in hospitals, nursing homes, and schools, as well as programs in non-institutionalized settings. As distinguished from AAA, animal-assisted therapy (AAT) refers to the use of an animal as a significant part of an individual treatment plan, typically conducted in a traditional therapy setting. As indicated, we further distinguish AAT (the use of actual animals) from the use of animal content or symbolic animals (puppets or drawings). AAT is particularly relevant to the treatment model of *AniCare Child*.

AAT is based on the observation, drawn from case studies and research findings, that the human-animal relationship can significantly affect human development (Beck & Katcher, 1996; Fine, 2000; Melson, 2001). For example, Poresky (1990, 1996) found that children with close relationships to their family pets scored higher on social competency and empathy measures. A one-year humane education program evaluated by Ascione (1992) found that children who participated in the program had higher mean scores for humane attitudes than the control group at the conclusion of the program and a year later. Corroborating Poresky's findings about the importance of the quality of the relationship, the researchers noted that "attitudes toward animals generalized to human-directed empathy — especially when the quality of the children's relations with their pets was considered as a covariate" (1996, p. 188). Looking at the effects of animals on human health, numerous research studies have demonstrated that a relationship with animals can have a salubrious effect on human health (Allen, 1996, 1998; Allen, Blascovich, Tomaka, & Kelsey, 1991; Beck & Katcher, 1996).

Research on companion animal therapy literature has not produced results as definitive as the research on the human-animal bond. In a 1984 review of the pet therapy literature, Beck and Katcher concluded that most of the research was descriptive or hypothesis-generating and that of six experimental studies on pet therapy, only one showed a measurable benefit of the presence of pets.

Since that review, several other papers have reviewed the literature in regard to the efficacy of AAT (Barba, 1995; Fine, 2010; Garrity & Stallone, 1998; Voelker, 1998). In the most comprehensive meta-analysis to date, Nimer and Lundhal (2007) found that AAT showed moderately improved outcomes in persons with autism, medical disabilities, behavioral problems, and poor well-being. The authors noted the need for more rigorous research to identify conditions and specific populations where AAT would be most effective. Garrity and Stallone (1998) report that only 5 of 25 studies applied appropriate experimental designs. Results from these papers suggest that there continues to be a need to provide more rigorous empirical evidence of the value of AAT with specific populations, including juveniles who abuse animals.

When working with children who commit animal abuse, safeguards need to be in place to ensure that their contact with animals is either highly supervised or denied. If AAT is involved, this simply means that the therapist must take precautions within the session. Close supervision is required and the type of animal chosen is an important consideration. For example, children who cannot control their aggression should not be placed near small animals, even under supervision. At all times, the animals' welfare needs to be a priority to ensure that they cannot be injured and that the interactions do not cause the animals stress or discomfort.

It is also the responsibility of the therapist to take measures, where possible, to assure the well-being of any animals with whom the client might come into contact. For example, the therapist might discuss the presence of a companion animal in the home with the parents of a child who has abused animals. (It should be noted that current governing laws and regulations do not protect the liability of a therapist who breaks client confidentiality to report animal abuse or a reasonable prospect of animal abuse.)

The case of a young Caucasian boy (below) illustrates the problem of managing client exposure to animals outside of the therapy. On two occasions in the course of his treatment, in reaction to recent losses he suffered, Calvin killed two street cats when he visited his foster mother.

Although additional research studies are needed to understand if and how AAT is effective in psychotherapy—and despite the necessity of closely monitoring the animal's welfare—the use of AAT has intuitive appeal. As we continually emphasize in *AniCare Child*, children's relationships with animals—whether one is actually present in the session, a puppet animal, or an animal reported by them—provide an important tool to the therapist. It aids in understanding the child and his or her functioning, is useful in treating the child, and helps the child to open up to the therapeutic process.

The power of animals to reach children when other approaches have failed is dramatically illustrated in the following report of an initial session with Ronald.

4.1.5 Clinical Case: Ronald

Ronald, an 8-year-old Caucasian boy, was referred by his school to treatment for aggressive behavior in school and for sexual gesturing—suggestive dancing and grabbing girls' buttocks. In addition to his aggressive and sexual misconduct, he also had abused and killed his cat. On one occasion he set the cat's tail on fire. At another time, he reacted angrily when the cat scratched him and threw the cat against the wall, killing her. In his neighborhood, there had been a number of animals who had been attacked by having firecrackers inserted in their rectums and then lit. Ronald's mother thought he was involved in those acts; however, he vigorously denied it.

Ronald was diagnosed as being hyperactive and began taking Ritalin. Although disruptive at school, he performed well and appeared to be bright.

He came to once-a-week treatment for a period of eight months, after which his mother withdrew him from treatment because she thought he had improved. The therapist also believed Ronald had made considerable progress; however, she did not believe that his treatment was complete.

Ronald's mother had no visible means of support and claimed to work sporadically; it was rumored that she was a prostitute. A variety of men passed through their home, many referred to as Ronald's "uncles." Ronald came from a large family, with fluid and transitory boundaries. His brothers, sisters, cousins, grandparents, and other relatives moved frequently and his household composition shifted at various times.

The relationship between Ronald and his mother was problematic. Although parents are required by the treating agency to participate in the therapy, she rarely came. Typically, she left Ronald for his appointment without coming in. At times she would drop him off long before the time of his appointment. His mother used switches to punish Ronald for his behavior. She also appeared to have unrealistic expectations of him and often seemed irritated by having to deal with him. At the beginning of treatment, when Ronald had to leave his therapy session, he would become aggressive and angry.

In Ronald's initial interview, he refused to talk to the therapist. Another therapist and her animal co-therapist, a dog named Rex, were invited to join the session in an attempt to get Ronald to respond. When they entered the therapy room, Ronald was out of sight, having climbed into a large toy box, where he lay curled up, refusing to talk or even to be seen.

The following interaction occurred as the therapist and Rex entered the room:

Therapist: *I hope there is no one here who is afraid of dogs. And I hope they don't mind being licked and sniffed. If they have any concerns they need to say something now! Ronald remained silent. Rex walked over to the box where Ronald was hiding and sniffed him. An arm emerged from the box; Rex licked his hand. Then a leg appeared, then another leg, and slowly Ronald unfolded from his hiding place.*

Ronald: *Oh my God! Look at that dog! What's his name?*

Therapist: *His name is Rex and he is a pet therapy dog. He works with kids like you to help them.*

Ronald: *I want to play with that dog! Can I?*

Therapist: *Well, you were sent to us because you were doing things that got you into trouble. And we will need to talk about those things and work on them.*

Ronald: *O.K. I will do that.*

Therapist: *We know that sometimes it is hard to talk to another person. I want you to know that Rex is a very good listener. He listens and I can act as his interpreter. Shall we go back to my room to talk?*

Ronald: *Yes, let's go!*

Therapist: *O.K. Why don't you ask Rex to come and he will go with you. Ronald led Rex back to their therapy room.*

4.1.6 Summary

There are many ways to connect to clients, and each therapist finds his or her own way to approach this task. *AniCare Child* has described being sensitive to one's own reactions as therapist, joining the client through the use of language, framing the therapy, and the direct and indirect use of animals as examples. Establishing and maintaining a connection underlies all other therapeutic tasks. A positive and trusting connection to the therapist provides a safe and secure foundation for the client to express feelings, explore problems, and experiment with change.

4.2 Empathy

If we take off our therapist hats for a moment and take a naïve look, empathy is really an amazing phenomenon. Although imperfectly, we are able to experience what other individuals are experiencing in a particular moment—to get into their shoes, to "see" from their point of view. Although in the end we always retain our own point of view, we are not fully stuck in our own perspective for it is readily and in an ongoing way informed by our empathic appreciation of other peoples' points of view.

Recent research has established a neurological basis for empathy. "Mirror neurons" are brain cells that are activated both when a person performs an intentional act and when he or she perceives someone else do the same act (Di Pellegrino, Fadiga, Fogassi, Gallese, & Rizzolatti, 1992). An observed behavior has an impact on us in some ways similar to that behavior when we do it ourselves. When I see you stub your toe, the same part of my brain is stimulated as when I stub my own.

As therapists, the ability to empathize has considerable value in our efforts to understand our clients—directly appreciating "where they are coming from" informs our theory and interventions. In some therapies, empathy is the primary posture of the therapist. It is also valuable, arguably invaluable, for the client to be able to empathize with others to better understand them and to form constructive relationships with them.

Some nonhuman mammals and some birds also have mirror neurons. In fact, they were first discovered in nonhuman primates. This has important implications for human-animal relationships and for the causes of and treatment of animal abuse. Animal abuse can be caused by a failure to empathize. Most cultures teach people not to empathize with animals in most contexts (e.g., the supermarket meat counter). However, empathy also can be used to exploit other individuals (e.g., brainwashing). *AniCare Child* capitalizes on the positive implications of empathy as a tool to form reciprocal and respectful relationships with both other humans and animals.

As with many other skills, there is considerable variation in individual ability based on differences in both constitution and socialization. The following two sections provide sets of skills both to identify and express one's own feelings and those of others and largely constitute an individual's emotional intelligence.

It is helpful to determine whether a client needs more help with empathy or self-management skills. The handbook begins with the section on empathy followed by one on self-management, but reversing this order may be appropriate, depending on the strengths and weakness of a client in these two areas and your judgment as to whether to begin with the area of strength or weakness. Many of the tools under the two Sects. 4.2 (pp. 33–55) and 4.3 (pp. 55–89) are flexible and, as will be noted, can be adapted for use in either or both types of corrective intervention.

Locating your client in the following 2 × 2 schema may be helpful:

Empathy

	Low	High
Low		
High		

Self-Management

4.2.1   Identifying and Expressing Feelings

In most instances, a client will need to be able to identify and express his or her own feelings before he can empathize with those of others. However, in some instances focusing on the feelings of others may be less threatening and more developed. The therapist's judgment and flexibility are important in determining the order of use of the interventions in this section and the following on "empathy development."

Many therapies recognize that thinking and feeling are dynamic and interrelated processes and therefore include a focus on helping the client express his or her feelings. Therapists with a psychodynamic approach devote particular attention to this aspect of therapy and emphasize the significance of the child's emotional life in the organization of her or his psychological structure. Some cognitive behavioral therapies, such as rational-emotive therapy, propose an intricate relationship between emotion, thought, and behavior. Ellis, the founder of rational-emotive therapy, stated that "Emotion, thought, and behavior rarely, if ever, are pure or unalloyed; each includes important elements of the others, and all three continually interact with and cause aspects of one another" (Ellis 1986, p. 278). As Ellis' comment suggests, expression of feelings entails multiple abilities—recognizing, identifying, owning, and regulating feelings—and entails cognitive, affective, and behavioral responses.

Children are more amenable to imaginative interventions; therefore, child therapists typically have many more techniques at their disposal than adult therapists.

Characterized as "play therapies," they include the use of toys and puppets, doll houses, drawing, coloring, and sand painting. Some techniques involve asking a child to complete the end of a story or to make up a story after looking at a picture.

From this panoply of techniques, *AniCare Child* presents the following techniques:

- Exercises to help children identify and positively address a number of feeling states
- A projective tool, the "Animals-at-Risk" TAT
- A clinical case example of the use of puppet role-play
- Therapist-facilitated expression, illustrated by a clinical case
- The use of animal-assisted therapy to foster attachment and encourage expression

The therapist must assess the client's current level of functioning in this area and, accordingly, adjust order, emphasis, and age-appropriateness.

Exercises

Throughout *AniCare Child* a number of exercises are offered. Therapists may use their own judgment to determine which exercises are age-appropriate for a particular child. These exercises also can be used with children in the context of individual or group treatment.

Two exercises, "Emotional Tracking" and "Emotional Choices," are for use with children to help them learn to identify and articulate a variety of feelings and emotional states. Learning the differences between emotions, such as sadness and depression, fear and anxiety, and anger and frustration, is important to the clinical process and the child's progress and treatment. "Emotional Tracking," which focuses mainly on helping the child differentiate among, his or her feelings, can be used over the course of therapy; therapists are encouraged to supplement and add to the exercise. "Emotional Choices," designed to encourage children to identify other beings' emotional states, builds on "Emotional Tracking." "Emotional Choices," with its focus on learning how others might be experiencing a situation, prepares the child for empathy development and problem-solving.

Emotional Tracking

Show the child "Emotional Tracking" diagram (p. 38) and say, "As we talk about different situations, show me which word or words best describe how the person is feeling." For younger children the diagram can be modified by replacing words with faces.

"Emotional Tracking" can be used with the situations described in "Emotional Choices" and can also be used throughout the course of therapy to educate the child about his or her feelings. For example, when exploring the events that preceded the animal abuse, have the child articulate what he or she was feeling at different moments. In a parallel discussion, ask the child to imagine how the animal was feeling. Children might resist this exercise initially and will have to be gently encouraged. At times, the therapist may have to assist the child by speaking for him or her.

Emotional Choices

Discuss the situations below and ask the child to imagine what it is like to be the person or animal in the circumstance described. Again, a child may have to be encouraged and helped to develop the ability to place himself or herself in another being's situation:

- Cary is walking home with his small dog. Some older boys walk by and make fun of him and his little dog, calling them both runts. How does Cary feel? How does he feel about his dog? What could he do?
- Jimmy pushes Tony around during recess and grabs his ball. When Tony tells Jimmy to stop he just laughs and yells, "baby, baby, baby!" How does Tony feel? What should he do?
- The teacher tells the class that whoever finishes their worksheet first can take an extra 5 minutes at recess. Karen leans over Sara's shoulder and begins copying from Sara's worksheet. Then Karen leaps up and says, "I'm finished first!" Sara knows Karen only finished first because she copied her work. How does Sara feel? What would you do if you were Sara?
- Sam comes home with a friend, Morty, to play on the computer. As soon as he walks in the door, his father yells at him in front of his friend because the family dog, Sophie, dug up one of the rose bushes in the backyard. His father tells Sam that Morty has to go home and he can't play computer games for two days. How does Sam feel? How does he feel about Sophie? How does Morty feel? Is there something Sam can do?
- Abdul comes from another country and only recently learned English, so he speaks with a noticeable accent. There are three boys in his classes who make fun of the way he talks. How do you think Abdul feels? What do you imagine his thoughts are? If you were Abdul, what would you do? If you saw students teasing Abdul, how would you react?
- Linda is new at her school. One day two girls whom she would like to be friends with ask her if she wants to walk home with them. She happily agrees. When they are walking home the girls find rocks to throw at squirrels. They are laughing and encouraging Linda to throw rocks, too. Linda pretends to pick up the rocks and throw them, but she doesn't really do it. One rock hits a squirrel and Linda can see it hurt him. What does she feel? What should she do? Should Linda say anything? To whom?
- The teacher has instructed the students in her class to raise their hand before talking. Hernando is always careful to do this, yet a lot of the other students don't wait and just call out the answer. Sometimes Hernando doesn't get a chance to talk. What do you think Hernando should do about this? How do you think he feels about this situation?

- Rusty is a friendly pit bull mix. He loves being around people. His caretaker, Mike, lives alone and spends a lot of time away from home with his friends and at work. He leaves Rusty tied in the backyard when he is gone. Rusty can hear people next door sometimes, and his tail wags in anticipation that he might get a visit. But no one comes. How do you think Rusty feels? What are his days and evenings like?

- Ann's family is poor and her clothes are old and look a little ragged. There are two girls who sit behind her in class and they spend a lot of time making fun of her. They whisper to one another, "Look at Raggedy Ann." How do you think Ann feels when they do this? If you were sitting nearby and heard them making fun of Ann, what would you do?

- Cal and Mike take a shortcut to school, crossing a wooded area. They notice two older boys tying a dog to a tree and kicking the dog. The boys, who are laughing, see them and call for them to come over. What do you think Cal and Mike feel? What should they do?

- Adam is Mrs. Clancy's cat. Adam is friendly and enjoys visiting some of his friends in the neighborhood. One day, three boys saw him sleeping by his front porch. They grabbed him, threw him in a cloth bag, and then began throwing the bag around, with Adam in it. How do you think Adam felt? What do you think he might have been thinking? How would Mrs. Clancy feel to know what is happening to Adam? If you saw the boys doing this, what would you do?

- Tammy is a mixed-breed dog who lives with her human family—a mother, father, Sara, a 10-year-old girl, and Jim, her 12-year-old brother. Tammy loves to take long walks with Sara and Jim. One day Tammy's family is away from home for a long time; they can't come home at their usual time. When Sara comes home, Tammy hears her even before she gets to the front door of the house. Tammy runs up to greet her, tail wagging, licking her on the face. Sara laughs, gives Tammy a quick hug, then gets her leash, puts it on her, and takes her for a walk in the neighborhood. How do you think Sara felt? How do you think Tammy felt?

Body Scan

Use "Emotional Tracking" to identify three feelings you would like to work on. Take one of those feelings and imagine having it. As you imagine the feeling, where do you feel it in your body? Does it have a particular quality? For example, does it move, or pulsate, or does it feel warm or cold? Do you "see" the feeling in your mind? How do you see it? Describe the feeling as completely as possible. Repeat these steps with the other two feelings you identified.

Emotional Diary

Use the following chart to record at least one important feeling you have each day. Do this every day for a week. By each feeling, make a note of what was happening at the time, and then what you did, if anything. Then think about what you did and note how you could have responded in another way. The first line gives an example of how to use the "Emotional Diary."

Emotional tracking

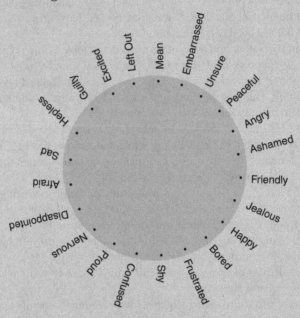

Emotional diary

Emotional Diary			
Feeling	**Situation**	**Response**	**Think About**
EX: Angry	My brother took my sweater.	I yelled at him.	I could offer to trade my sweater for his hat.

Projective Tools: The "Animals-at-Risk" Thematic Apperception Test

The "Animals-at-Risk" TAT (Lockwood, 1983, 1985) presents drawings of scenes involving children, companion animals, and sometimes an adult (Appendix C, pp. 92–99). They are intended to encourage discussion of events in the family, particularly those that create tension in the human-animal relationship. Therapists use the "Animals-at-Risk" TAT to explore children's attitudes toward and experience with animals and to uncover incidents in the family and elsewhere that influenced their relationship with animals. (See pp. 67–68 for instructions on how to administer the instrument in a broader therapeutic context). The "Animals-at-Risk" TAT can also help the child clarify his or her thoughts and feelings and sort through previous experiences. As a projective instrument, the pictures are designed to be ambiguous and provocative and are more likely to evoke emotional responses than direct questioning.

"Self-management Skills: Projective Techniques" (Demonstration DVD, Treatment submenu) illustrates the use of the Animals-at-Risk TAT in the context of an ongoing treatment (with Amanda).

Puppet Role-Play

To illustrate the usefulness of puppet role-play, we present an extended clinical case of therapy with Tony, a 7-year-old boy who, with his 9-year-old friend, Kenneth, had been referred by the courts for animal abuse. For the therapist working with Tony, puppet role-play is an important tool for treating children who abuse animals. In her practice, she maintains a variety of animal puppets of different sizes and species, and puppets of people as well.

Clinical Case: Tony

Background

Tony, along with Kenneth, used a pit bull to attack and kill a rabbit. The boys stole a rabbit, Velvet, from a neighbor, and tied her by the legs upside down from a tree. They then jumped over a fence, released another neighbor's pit bull from his cage, and took the dog to the location where they had tied the rabbit. Kenneth commanded the dog to attack the rabbit, which the animal did, killing Velvet.

Kenneth, the instigator of the attack, had approached Tony with the idea. After Kenneth stole the rabbit, he instructed Tony to jump a neighbor's fence and release the pit bull. Tony did this, and the pit bull obeyed Tony, who did not have a leash or any other means to control the dog, except by voice command. Kenneth and Tony staged the attack in a field that was located in the middle of their neighborhood. The guardian of the rabbit contacted the police after neighbors informed her of what had happened.

The investigating officer was a member of a "link coalition," a grassroots team comprising the local Police Department, Fire Department, Animal Care Division, Municipal Courts, Criminal Justice Program, the Treatment Center, and many other agencies. The team works together to identify people at risk, develop intervention strategies, open lines of communication, and share information. Both boys were arrested and ticketed by the officer. He also brought charges of negligence against the guardian of the pit bull, who had been suspected of animal fighting. The man fled the state before he could be charged and a bench warrant was issued for his arrest.

The case went to Municipal Court, where in addition to being fined and placed on one year's probation, Tony and Kenneth were ordered to receive counseling. At first, the woman who was the guardian of the rabbit said she would not press charges if the boys would go to church. When they didn't agree to her request, she pressed charges. The arresting officer recommended treatment for them. The judge concurred and required the boys to attend 12–14 individual counseling sessions. The boys also were required to report to a probation officer once a month, who would oversee their conduct and determine whether they were meeting the terms of their probation. The therapist sent monthly reports to the probation department. If the therapist determined that her court-ordered clients need more treatment, she would notify the court of that assessment. In her experience, the court has responded to her recommendations for further treatment. The boys' families paid for the treatment on a sliding fee scale.

While on probation, the court ordered the two boys not to have any contact with one another. However, the boys attend the same school and walk to school on a similar route, so it is not clear whether the terms of the probation were being followed.

The therapist describes Kenneth as the brighter, more articulate, and creative of the two. He is an adept prevaricator, able to adapt his story to the interviewer's questions. At times his ability to fabricate self-protective explanations is quite skillful, temporarily inducing the interviewer to believe him. Kenneth also gives the appearance of being tough. He has adopted a swaggering walk and speaks in a "tough" tone. Kenneth appears alert, "sharp-eyed," and is able to read a social situation.

In contrast, Tony, who is small for his age, appears vulnerable. Unlike Kenneth, he is not a very good manipulator. He may attempt self-protective deception, but cannot sustain it. He is compliant, even submissive, around authority figures. He does not talk in the presence of his mother and hangs his head, mute, when she is by his side. Tony does not appear aggressive and often becomes tearful and distressed when he is talking about his situation.

Kenneth appeared to have cultivated the relationship with Tony with a design to influence a younger confederate. The therapist believes that Tony responded to him out of a need for attachment and attention.

Previous Treatment

Neither boy had been in treatment before. Kenneth has been in trouble at school. His behavioral difficulties include being charged with petty theft, talking back to teachers, taking another child's jacket, and being aggressive with other children. Tony did not display aggressive behavior in school, although teachers reported that he frequently came to school unprepared and without his homework. Tony was aware of Kenneth's theft of the jacket but did not report it.

Family/Education/Social Background

Tony and Kenneth, who are African-American, live in a poor, lower-middle-class neighborhood, scarred by frequent violence. Both boys have been exposed to repeated violence and dogfighting is common in their neighborhood. Training apparatus used to train dogs for fights, pit bulls, and other signs of animal fighting are common sights. "Street fighting," because it is spontaneous and doesn't occur in a fixed location, often eludes law enforcement unless there are strong animal abuse laws that permit arrests based on evidence other than witnessing a fight, such as scarred animals and training gear. Both boys were apparently exposed to sexual activity, as both have knowledge of explicit sexual acts far beyond what one would expect for children their ages.

Tony lives with his mother, who is a day-care provider. Tony lived with his mother, father, and two older half-siblings, a sister and a brother, until he was 5 years old. His father, to whom he was attached, had an affair with another woman and his mother left their family home in Santa Fe and moved to another state with Tony. He has not had contact with his father or siblings since that time. After Tony's father learned about his son's arrest and treatment, he sought custody and visitation rights. The mother, suspicious of the father's intentions, is blocking the father's efforts to make contact with Tony.

Tony's mother treats him harshly. She chastises him in public, berates him, takes privileges and toys away from him, and whips him with belts and other devices on occasion as a means of punishing him. After revealing to his therapist that his mother had beaten him, the therapist reported the incident to the local children's services agency. The agency investigated the report but concluded that it did not have enough evidence of child abuse to continue. At the same time, the therapist observed the mother caressing Tony's back in a somewhat sexualized manner, referring to him as her "little man."

Kenneth lives at home with his mother, father, and two older brothers. His father is a semiskilled worker and his mother is a homemaker. His mother says she supports his treatment and has made some attempts to comply with the therapist's suggestions. For example, the parents were told to bar their children from watching any violent activities—videos, television, movies, computer games—since this seemed to stimulate their aggression. Kenneth's mother could adhere to this advice for a period of time, but eventually Kenneth would gain access again to these activities.

Kenneth's father abuses alcohol, is a strict disciplinarian, and uses harsh, physical punishment on his children. His father was arrested six years ago for child abuse following an incident in which a neighbor heard him hitting the children and reported him to the police. Reportedly, the father tried to intimidate other family members by choking the family pet. This report, however, was not substantiated. He does not participate in treatment. The older brothers have also had trouble in school and with the law.

Relationships with Other Animals

Tony had a dog to whom he was very close; however, his mother gave the dog away about a year before the incident (and about 6 months after his mother left his father). Tony was inconsolable. When Tony's mother became aware of his distress, she tried to retrieve Tony's dog but was not successful.

As noted earlier, Kenneth had caused minor injuries to the family cat and dog and had maimed a classroom hamster and turtle under his care for the weekend. He expressed no interest in the family pets and did not appear to be attached to them.

Using Puppet Role-Play

The therapist often uses human and animal puppets as a role-play technique. From a variety of puppets, the child chooses one to represent the animal victim and others to represent other affected parties, such as the human guardian of the victim and the child himself. The purposes of the puppet role-play are (1) to assist the child in expressing and identifying feelings, (2) to connect feelings with actions, (3) to learn alternative ways of responding, and (4) to facilitate the development of the child's empathic capacity.

In the present case, we are highlighting the particular usefulness of the technique in helping Tony to identify his feelings toward his mother. As noted earlier, his mother was a harsh disciplinarian and used physical force, verbal abuse, and public humiliation to control Tony. Tony adapted to this type of parenting by remaining mute, with his head downcast in the presence of his mother or other authorities. As the following descriptions of using puppet role-play illustrate, Tony was able to express his fear and sadness at his mother's harsh treatment of him and to accept comfort from the therapist. Tony had identified a bird puppet as his "special buddy." The following interaction occurred using the bird puppet.

Therapist: *Mom is yelling at us again. I feel bad about that.*
Tony: *(softly crying)*
Therapist: *(as the bird puppet) Let me give you a hug.*

Tony responded by leaning into her, almost crawling into her lap. He clutched the bird puppet against his chest, with the therapist's hand still in the puppet.

Tony, who has a fairly limited vocabulary, typically did not verbalize much. He might say, when role-playing with the puppets, that "Mom doesn't like me," or "I'm no good," or "I'm a bad boy." Speaking for the bird puppet, the therapist would reply, "I don't think you're a bad boy. I like who you are."

In these instances, Tony's participation in the puppet role-playing allowed him to express his sorrow about his mother's treatment of him and to experience another person's concern for him. Through his interaction with the therapist and the puppets, Tony was able to experience sadness that previously he had not been able to articulate. Through the experience of that sadness with a responsive therapist, he was able to tolerate the feeling. The therapist believes that by learning to cope with his sorrow about his mother's treatment of him, Tony laid the groundwork for learning about the way in which sorrow shaped his life, including his vulnerability to Kenneth's attention and influence.

Therapist-Facilitated Expression

At times the child may not be able to acknowledge threatening feelings, such as shame, guilt, and anxiety. Children who commit egregious acts of animal abuse may be more likely to experience threatening feelings once they understand the gravity of their actions. In these cases, the therapist may facilitate the child's expression, speaking for the child and acknowledging actions and feelings that the child cannot. Susan Krinsk has observed that some children cannot take direct responsibility for particular behaviors. She believes that, at times, the child does not have the emotional capacity to process or structure the various feelings and thoughts that would arise if certain behaviors were acknowledged. The same response in adults, however, might cause her concern; in fact, she remarked that if the adults she saw in treatment remained in denial she would refuse to continue the therapy.

Abused children often suffer from expressive language difficulties, and it may be more difficult for them to articulate their emotions. Whether a child has a temporary reluctance to express difficult feelings, is incapable of doing so, or simply will not, it is important for the therapist to address important feelings so that the child learns to acknowledge and express them.

Clinical Case: Ronald

The therapist approached Ronald, the 8-year-old boy referred for aggressive behavior in the classroom, a number of times with questions or statements about his cat, whom he had injured, then killed. Although she made numerous attempts such as "I wonder what happened to your cat?" or "Tell me what happened to your cat?" he refused to answer or even to acknowledge that the question had been asked. Completely closed down, the therapist believed that he felt too guilty to acknowledge what he had done. She compared his reaction to other children, some of whom could talk more easily about their animal abuse because they felt little or no remorse.

Since Ronald's demonstrated difficulty acknowledging the abuse he committed, the therapist addressed the issue by speaking for him.

Therapist: *I have heard some things about you and the cat you used to have. If these things occurred — if you hurt the cat — I am thinking about how the cat must have felt. I bet the cat must have felt so betrayed. And I bet the cat was really scared. And I think the cat also was probably confused, sad, and angry. Do you wonder how the cat felt? Do you think the cat might have felt this way—betrayed, and so scared, and very confused, and sad?*

Ronald: *(no answer, but he sat quietly and listened attentively with a somber mood)*

The therapist took time asking the questions, allowing for pauses and quiet between them. She adopted a receptive attitude toward Ronald, carefully observing him and gauging his reactions.

The therapist used the "therapist-facilitated expression" technique a number of times with Ronald throughout the treatment. At other times, when she brought up the cat, she would say the following:

Therapist: *I remember talking about your cat, and how you hurt her. We were wondering what the cat felt like. I also wonder how the cat's mom would have felt to see what happened to her cat. Or if the cat had babies, how would they have felt to see what happened? I imagine they would be frightened and sad. Can you imagine that?*

Ronald: *(no verbal response, but listening attentively)*

Therapist: *When I get mad I may feel like kicking, and hitting, and throwing, too. What if I kicked Rex? How would I feel if I did that? Rex wouldn't like it. It would hurt him. And he certainly doesn't deserve it. And he would feel confused that I had done that to him, since he relies on me and trusts me. And I know I would feel really bad about myself. It would be horrible to feel that way. I wonder if that is how you feel about hurting your cat.*

Animal-Facilitated Attachment and Expression

Frequently it is in and through the relationship with a therapist that a child will find the resources to confront painful memories and affect. For most clients, forming a trusting relationship or making a connection is a prerequisite for effective therapeutic work. In the extended case presented next, Susan Brooks demonstrates how a young boy learned to acknowledge and then regulate painful feelings through his attachment to her. Note how the therapist uses therapist-facilitated and animal-facilitated expression in tandem to help this client work through his complex and deep-seated attachment issues.

Clinical Case: Calvin[1]

Calvin came to Green Chimneys, a residential treatment program specializing in the care of children with emotional and behavioral needs. The 102 resident children and adolescents and the 30-day students share the rural environment with barnyard animals, domestic companion animals, and wildlife. The animals have been an integral part of the therapeutic milieu for more than 50 years.

Calvin was admitted to Green Chimneys at the age of 9, when he began seeing Brooks one hour a week for two and a half years. During the termination period, Calvin attended 30-minute sessions twice a month for another year. He was discharged at age 13.

Family History

Calvin's mother had a long history of drug abuse and he was removed from her care. His father was in prison. He lived with his maternal grandmother, great-aunt, and 24-year-old cousin. Calvin's behavior, which seemed to worsen when he lived with his cousin, included crying, tantrums, head banging, rocking, and hyperactivity. He fought, bit, and threw objects at peers.

Assessment

His admitting diagnosis according to the DSM-III-R was "Axis I—Dysthymia and Conduct Disorder, Undifferentiated." Aggression to animals was not noted at the time.

The WISC-RIII showed Calvin to be a concrete thinker with a full-scale IQ of 97, which is in the average range.

Brooks reported that "The initial clinical formulation, documented by our admitting treatment team, centered around his suffering from early deprivation and neglect. It was felt that his capacity for meaningful relationships had been impaired. His mother's addiction and, hence, the loss of her emotionally and the loss of his father created emotional fragility and deep feelings of rejection, loss, and abandonment" (Ascione, Kaufmann, & Brooks, 2000, p. 346).

---

[1] Excerpts from "Animal Abuse and Developmental Psychopathology, Part IV (c) Case Study" by Ascione et al. (2000), reproduced by permission of the publisher.

Compounding Calvin's difficulties with abandonment and loss, he had three different social workers while at Green Chimneys. No one in his extended family would care for him, and yet they also rejected adoption.

After hitting a baby calf so hard that the calf went into a seizure, Calvin was sent to treatment.

Treatment

Brooks increased Calvin's time on the farm from 30 minute to 90 minutes a week. He worked alongside an intern who supervised him. Brooks wanted to observe how Calvin behaved with animals and how his response to animals might provide insight into his emotional life and reasoning.

At the beginning of the treatment, Brooks and Calvin would walk around the farm and Calvin would verbally provoke every living creature he came across. In a hyperactive manner, he cursed and talked about how he would kill or mutilate them. He told Brooks, "If no one was here, I'd kill all the animals except Duke and Doc." He never explained why he exempted the two draft horses from his imaginary mutilations. As Brooks observed, "Calvin was a bundle of rage." Brooks had to prepare herself for being around this unremittingly raging boy. In time, she sensed that Calvin felt accepted by her and they were able to engage in other activities other than walking around the farm. Calvin continued, however, to express verbal aggression toward more animals during those early sessions.

Brooks began to work with a 2-week-old rooster, Sebastian, who had been brought to live in a fish tank in Brooks' office for his safety. The parallels between the rooster's abandonment and Calvin's initiated many helpful therapeutic interactions. Brooks told the rooster things she wanted Calvin to hear and learn about Calvin through interactions with the rooster. Calvin was attracted to the rooster and initially personalized and misinterpreted some of the rooster's behavior. For example, when the rooster pecked him, Calvin thought Sebastian was purposely trying to hurt him. Brooks explained that Sebastian might be pecking out of fear, curiosity, or wanting to investigate a surface. Calvin developed an attachment to the rooster and was allowed to leave his classroom every day for a few minutes to check on him. Building on his successful attachment to Sebastian, Brooks introduced other animals to Calvin. Two important animal therapists at this time were Tinkerbell, a cockatiel, and Erika, a guinea pig. Working with these animals, Brooks helped Calvin understand how people and animals responded to him and how his responses affected them. Brooks would instruct Calvin to locate a feeling in his body and to get an image of the feeling in his heart region, head, neck, or whole body. He was then instructed to let the feeling travel down his arm into the animal. Calvin would pay attention to how the animal experienced the feeling. Erika and Tinkerbell might move away, tense up, snuggle, or allow Calvin to rub the back of their heads.

Calvin, who especially loved birds, began to see that his behavior toward animals had a lot to do with how they responded to him. He realized his tenseness turned them away and he began to see parallels between his interactions with the animals and his relationships with peers in the dormitory.

Although Calvin exhibited interest in animals, he regressed when he visited a potential foster mother. While there, he stomped a kitten to death because she had "bothered" him. This incident occurred one week after his first social worker left him. Calvin was unable to understand the connection between his feelings about the social worker's departure, his mother's and father's abandonment of him, and his violence toward the kitten. After this incident, Calvin responded angrily toward other staff and peers. He also placed hand lotion in the bowl of the dormitory dog, who ate it and became sick. At the same time, there were moments when Calvin was observed to be quiet and gentle with animals during his job and during farm class time.

However, Calvin showed no remorse for hurting the dog or for his aggressive behavior toward his peers. As a result, he was barred from farm jobs and therapeutic riding classes for two weeks, which were activities that he valued. Brooks and the staff discussed with Calvin his feelings about not being able to come to the farm and suggested parallels between his feelings and the feelings he had inflicted on the dog.

When working with the farm animals, Calvin received immediate feedback from Brooks or a staff member about his progress in dealing with his anger. He slowly began to master his aggression and to integrate what he learned from working with the animals, showing a greater tolerance for painful emotional states. At one point, Calvin was able to articulate, "I feel better when I hurt an animal." Brooks saw this as a turning point. By articulating a feeling, Calvin was learning to hold it internally, rather than respond to the urge to act on it. He came to learn that he hurt animals in order to get rid of his painful feelings. He made the animal suffer so that he would not.

Despite his progress and his growing attachment to Brooks and many of the animals, feelings of abandonment would overwhelm him. When Brooks gave Calvin five weeks' notice that she would be away for six weeks, Calvin killed another cat at his potential foster mother's house. He refused to meet with Brooks directly in a session, would yell at Brooks across campus, follow her and swear at her. Brooks continued to try to make contact with Calvin, who refused it. When Calvin was directly expressing his rage at Brooks, there were no incidents of inflicting harm on animals.

Upon Brooks' return, Calvin resumed talking angrily about wanting to hurt animals. Brooks observed that Calvin had killed the cat because he was not able to say how angry he was that she had gone away. Calvin would make aggressive movements toward an animal, then laugh as the animal avoided him. Brooks worked on having Calvin express the feeling, "I'm angry," rather than act on it by threatening an animal.

Calvin then suffered additional losses. He learned that his parents' rights had been terminated and that he had siblings from his biological mother who were living with his maternal grandmother. Feeling rejected, he directed his rage at female staff members and teachers. A short time after that, another social worker left. His relationship with Brooks, Erika, the guinea pig, and Tinkerbell, the cockatiel, seemed to comfort him. Snuggling Erika in his lap, Calvin asked Brooks to read a story to him. Tinkerbell came in and sat quietly on his shoulder. When Brooks discussed the idea of sharing feelings, Calvin said that his animals realized he was sad and were reaching out to him. Brooks and Calvin discussed trust and what that felt like.

Calvin continued to successfully interact with the animals. Walking Joe the ferret on a leash, he learned to respond to the ferret's actions and wishes, rather than his own. Feeding wild coyotes, he learned that suspicious animals could learn to trust him. With Peaches, the parrot, who was sensitive to his energy, he understood he had to earn her trust in order to enjoy a relationship with her.

Brooks again told Calvin that she would be leaving on vacation for 6 weeks. This time Calvin said, "So long this time like last time?" This time Calvin was able to talk about his anger. Although he refused to come to the next therapy session, Brooks went to his classroom and together they found on the globe the country she was going to visit. Brooks also gave Calvin a picture of Tinkerbell, himself, and her to keep while he was away. She sent him a postcard, telling Calvin when she would return.

While Brooks was gone, Calvin had episodes in which he was verbally aggressive, but he did not harm any animals. Upon her return, he initially refused to see her and told Brooks how angry he was at her. When Brooks opened her arms to Calvin, he approached her and allowed himself to be hugged.

As Calvin entered the termination phase, he began work with another parrot, Lorita, who bit him one day. He began to cry but made no attempt to hurt her. Brooks discussed his response with him, noting how far he had come in not trying to hurt the bird. Calvin said he understood that she was "just afraid."

In summary, the therapeutic goal of expression is to help the child learn to identify and acknowledge feelings, some of which are painful—shame, guilt, abandonment. Through that process, the child integrates those feelings and feeling states into his or her psychological structure, learns to modulate them, and begins to use feelings as sources of important information about which to make decisions. Instead of the child being controlled by feelings, the child learns to identify, understand, and use feelings for positive ends.

4.2.2 Empathy Development

There are many other activities and interventions that are designed to develop empathy. One of the most effective ways to foster empathy is for the therapist to convey empathy for the child. In addition, the therapist's expectations that the child can improve his or her empathic abilities will encourage the child to do so.

Increasingly, clinicians as well as educators are recognizing the importance of encouraging the development of empathy. They recognize, as Shapiro stated, that "while it does not promise ethical treatment, empathy can be the basis of an ethic of respect and compassion" (Shapiro 1990, p. 47).

Affect or "feeling with" the other is the central component of empathy, but it also involves cognitive processes as all feelings have some at least implicit meaning. Sympathy, described as "feeling for" the other, is closely related to empathy and often is a consequence of it. Sympathy, which involves a desire to alleviate the other's distress, is most closely related to altruistically motivated prosocial behaviors (Eisenberg & Strayer, 1987).

The capacity for empathy develops with the experience of having one's own emotional needs satisfied, something many therapists realize is an important ingredient of treatment. In addition, empathy is developed within the context of social experience, including psychotherapy. Empathy, then, is a capacity that can be learned and developed in most individuals. It is an important motivator for prosocial behavior and contributes to moral judgment and actions.

Presumably, children who are in treatment for animal abuse have had empathic failures. Although their empathic failures were in relationship to animals, one could assume that they also had deficiencies in feeling empathy in other situations. The background of children with striking lapses of empathy and who committed severe acts of animal abuse should be assessed to ascertain if they have been abused and, if so, how severely.

Empathy can be encouraged through a variety of means. In *AniCare Child*, we present three approaches to empathy development:
- Psychosocial-emotional exercises
- Puppet role-play
- Animal-assisted therapy

The following exercises are intended to help the client develop empathy, particularly for animals. Before using, make sure the client is ready for them. If clients can identify a variety of feelings as ascertained by their facility with the four exercises in the Identifying and Expressing Feelings subsection (pp. 34–39), which focus on feelings about self, they can move on to these exercises or, if more appropriate, the use of puppet role-play or animal-assisted therapy.

The approach suggested in the exercises begins with empathizing with other children, then with animals, and finally with abused animals. For some clients, you may need to supplement whichever of the three approaches you use by sequencing materials so that the client is presented with objects of empathy in the following order:
- A human friend in a positive situation
- A human friend in a negative situation
- An animal friend in a positive situation
- An animal friend in a negative situation
- The animal(s) that the client abused

Exercises

Read the story to the child or have the child read it aloud. Explore the child's reaction to the story, using the discussion questions as a guide. Note that in the exercise "New Kid at School" the questions are asked at three different points in the story.

Empathizing with People

First Day at School

Meredith is 5 years old and it is her first day at school. As she and her mother walk up to the school, she is walking so slowly that her mother has to gently tug her along to keep her walking. She won't go in the door and her mother has to carry her in. She has her arms wrapped tightly around her mother's shoulders and she won't look up at the teachers who are smiling at her, trying to encourage her to say hello.

Discussion: How do you think Meredith is feeling? What makes you think that? Have you ever felt like that? What would help her feel better?

Play Ball

Kevin loved to play baseball, but he didn't always do well. Sometimes he dropped the ball or didn't see it when it was thrown to him. He was a little better at batting. Kevin saw some boys at the end of the playground who were starting to play ball. He knew some of them from his school. As he walked toward them, he called out, "Hey, can I play with you?" They looked at him and laughed. A couple of the boys said, "You got to be kidding, butterfingers!"

Discussion: How do you think Kevin felt? What different feelings do you imagine he had as he approached the boys? How did he feel when they laughed and called him "butterfingers"? Why do you think the boys responded that way to Kevin? What were they feeling? How might they have treated Kevin differently? What should Kevin do now?

The New Kid at School

Even though it is the middle of the year, today is John's first day at his school. He and his family just moved to their neighborhood, so John had to go to a new school. As John waits for the school bus, he sees other kids who are starting to gather. He looks at them but they don't say anything. Then they get on the bus. The other kids are kidding around with one another, laughing, and pushing into one another. John tries to smile at one of the kids closest to him, but nobody seems to notice him.

Discussion: How do you think John feels? How would you feel at your first day in a new school?

When John gets to school, he is assigned to a seat in his first class. He notices a girl in the class who looks different from the rest of the students. Some of the other students seem to laugh at her as they walk by her desk. After class, she approaches John, says hello to him, and asks him if he is new in town.

Discussion: How should John respond to this girl? What do you think will happen if he is friendly to her? If he does not respond to her, how will she feel?

John smiles at the girl and tells her that he is a new student at school. When he asks her name, she says, "My name is Henrietta, but you won't hear that name used around here. A lot of the kids make fun of me by calling me 'hennyhenny, cluck cluck'." "Why do they do that?" John asks. Henrietta shrugs her shoulders and says, "I don't know. My family doesn't have much money and I just think they don't like me because I don't dress like them. But we can't afford it. I just try to avoid them." John answered, "That must be pretty hard to do since you go to school with them!"

Later when John is walking down the hall, a bunch of kids approach him and say, "Hey, new boy, I saw you talking to 'hennyhenny, cluck cluck.' Are you a chicken too?"

Discussion: What should John do now? How do you think he feels? What thoughts are going through his mind?

John laughs at the group of kids and says, "Nothing wrong with being a chicken...at least chickens and their families certainly feel that way. But, no, my name is John Garth and this is my first day at school. My family and I moved from the southern part of the state. What are your names? Do any of you belong to any school clubs? Could you tell me about them?"

Discussion: What do you think happens now? How do you think John feels? How do the other boys feel about him?

Empathizing with Animals

Fallen Bird

A very little baby bird was in her nest, waiting for her mother and father to return with food. She was eager to see them so she wiggled to the edge of the nest. But she made a mistake, went too far, and fell out of the nest. She landed on the ground below the tree, all alone. She didn't know how to get back to her nest because she was too young to fly.

Discussion: If you were the baby bird, how would you feel? Would you feel alone? Frightened? Sad? What do you imagine it was like for her to fall from her nest? Picture her in your mind and how she is feeling as she found herself alone on the ground. Can you describe what is going through her mind? What she feels like inside? What do you think will happen next? If you saw her on the ground, what would you do?

Family Dog

Toby is a small dog in a large family where there often is a lot of fighting and screaming. The mother and father yell at one another, especially the dad. Sometimes he bangs his fist on the counter. There are three kids: Alice is 6 years old, Tim is 8 years old, and Jerry just turned 10 years of age. The Dad also yells a lot at the kids, and sometimes he slaps the boys on their backsides or shakes them a little when he is angry. Toby gets yelled at also. Tim tries to protect her by taking her into his room when there is a lot of yelling, but he can't always do that. One night when his dad came home late and dinner wasn't ready, he really blew his top. He banged his fist on the table so hard that the dishes fell on the floor and broke. Toby was under the table at the time. As she tried to run into another room, the father pushed her with his foot.

Discussion: What do you think it is like to be the family dog in this family? How would you feel if you were Toby under that table? Imagine yourself as Toby running from underneath the table. What feelings would you have? What do you think it is like for Alice, Tim, and Jerry, the three children? Do you think they have some of the same feelings as Toby?

Horse Trade

Sam was an old horse who pulled carriages in a large city. He had been doing this for a number of years, and the years of work on hot, hard pavements were beginning to show. His coat wasn't as shiny as it should have been and his legs were getting stiffer and stiffer from the stress of walking on hard surfaces and carrying heavy loads. One particular summer day, when it was very, very hot, Sam was walking very slowly. There were a number of passengers in the carriage and they were jumping around.

Ari, a man who owned a store on the route that Sam and his carriage took, was standing outside his store. He saw Sam pass by, pulling the carriage, and he noticed how slowly the horse was moving and how rapidly he was breathing. Ari had been thinking about Sam's age and condition for a while. He had meant to talk to Jake, the man who owned the carriage. Ari decided that this was the day to say something. He approached Sam's owner, Jake, who was sitting on top of the carriage and said, "When are you going to retire that old horse? He seems ready. I have an idea for you. I know a place that will take Sam where he can live and have access to a pasture and other horses. And I need a driver for a new delivery route I am about to start for my business. Why don't you retire Sam and drive for me?"

It didn't take Jake long to think about it; he eagerly agreed. The next day Ari took Sam to his new home and watched as Sam walked easily in the grassy lawn of the pasture and started to nuzzle the other horses there in greeting.

Discussion: What do you think it was like for Sam to be a carriage horse? How do you think he felt about it? Can you imagine that Sam had feelings as he pulled his carriage through the streets? What were they? Imagine being Sam and seeing the pasture for the first time. Can you describe what that was like for Sam? Think of the different sounds, sights, smells, and sensations and compare life being a carriage horse to a horse in a pasture with other horses. How did Sam feel when he met the other horses? Why do you think Ari did that for Sam and Jake?

Empathizing with Abused Animal(s)

From a Victim's Point of View[2]

Have the child write or describe what she or he did from the victim's point of view. (The therapist may help younger children with writing or have the

---

[2] These exercises were adapted from Cunningham and MacFarlane (1996).

child dictate the story.) Ask the child to imagine that she or he is the victim and to describe as completely as possible what it was like to be the animal victim: what sensations the animal felt, what feelings, what thoughts the animal had, how the animal reacted, and what the animal would say to the child now if he or she could. Some children may not be able to do this easily, and the therapist may have to provide prompts and encouragement. In some cases, the therapist may have to initially act for the child, writing or speaking for the animal victim. This exercise is not advised at the beginning of treatment, but at some point when a strong therapeutic alliance has been established and some progress had been made.

Letter of Apology[2]

Have the child write a letter of apology to the victim. In this letter, the therapist helps the child develop ways in which he or she can make amends. The letter should be specific and personal and might include how the writer feels now, what happened, why it happened, and who was responsible. The letter also should express concern for the victim and offer some kind of restitution. No restitution to the victim would be possible if the child killed the animal; however, the child could make restitution to animals of that species or to the human companions of the victim animal. Again, depending on the age of the child, the therapist may help the child write the letter.

Puppet Role-Play

Puppet role-play can be used to develop the capacity for empathy and to promote expression, as described earlier. For example, Tony's work with puppets had enabled him to feel more comfortable in identifying and expressing his feelings. After his experience with puppet role-play, Tony was willing to talk about his feelings of remorse for his role in the rabbit's death and to begin to identify with another creature's perspective. Building on this capacity, the therapist directed Tony to select puppets to represent Velvet, the rabbit who had been killed, Velvet's human guardian, and one for himself, the pit bull, and Kenneth. Tony then selected a puppet to play the abused rabbit.

Clinical Case: Tony

Therapist: *Tony, can you describe your personality to me? Show me what kind of voice you have?*
Tony: *(whispering lightly) I am a little rabbit, with soft fur and a soft voice.*
Therapist: *What are your favorite things to do?*
Tony: *I like carrots.*
Therapist: *I bet you do. What else do you like to do?*
Tony: *Play with my friends.*

The therapist continued to encourage Tony to talk about himself as the rabbit and ask him questions about his preferences, concerns, and his family. Once Tony had exhibited a capacity to "talk for the rabbit," the therapist began to inquire about the incident.

Therapist: *What would the rabbit say about what happened to her?*
Tony: *(crying) I didn't do anything. I don't understand why those boys were so mean to me.*
Therapist: *You sound confused; why did this happen?*
Tony: *Right. I'm a good rabbit.*
Therapist: *What are you thinking or feeling?*
Tony: *I wonder why no one will come to help me.*
Therapist: *Does that make you sad?*
Tony: *Yes, and scared.*
Therapist: *Yes, sad and scared. I'm very sorry for you rabbit.*
Tony: *Thank you. I don't want to be hurt.*
Therapist: *And no one should hurt you.*

The therapist reinforced the gains that Tony made in the role-playing interactions by pointing out to him that he learned to identify what he was feeling. She emphasized how important that was so he could understand what made him do certain things and so he could make better decisions. The therapist also reflected that he was learning about how others felt, including the animals that had gotten hurt.

The therapist's use of puppet role-play with Tony also helped him with problem-solving and to develop an awareness of his tendency to be manipulated by an older child. At the initial intake, Tony said that if he saw someone hurting an animal he would never tell anyone. After using puppet play to problem-solve this kind of situation, Tony said that if he saw someone abusing an animal, he would immediately leave the situation, find the nearest home, and ask them to call the police.

Animal-Assisted Therapy

Actual animals, as distinguished from puppets, also teach children empathy. Children with close bonds with pets have higher empathy scores (Poresky, 1990), and humane education programs have been shown to increase children's level of empathy (Ascione, 1992). Incorporating animals into the therapeutic process provides important opportunities for teaching empathy.

The following is another illustration of the therapist's work with Ronald, the young boy who had been sent to treatment for inappropriate sexual behavior (pp. 31–32). This clinical vignette vividly depicts the attraction that many children have for animals and how that affinity can be used to advance the therapeutic process and to develop empathy.

Clinical Case: Ronald

On occasion, Ronald would act too rough with Rex or would ignore Rex's desire to be left alone. The therapist always intervened to ensure Rex's well-being and safety. Rex would also let her know when he no longer liked a situation. If Rex did not feel comfortable with the interaction or was simply tired of it, he would move away, often lying underneath a desk in the room. Other times, Rex would stare at the therapist with his ears back, which she had learned from past experience was a signal that Rex wanted her to step in.

When Ronald acted inappropriately with Rex, the therapist used those moments to teach him about victim empathy and boundaries. This is illustrated in the following interaction in which Ronald was sitting next to Rex on the floor and then got up and tried to lie on top of Rex. Rex began shifting, clearly not enjoying Ronald's attention.

Therapist: *Ronald, Rex is giving me one of those looks. He is not enjoying having you try to lie on him.*

Ronald: *Why not?*

Therapist: *Sometimes dogs and people don't like it when someone gets too close to them. They want some space; they need some boundaries between themselves and the other person. My guess is that this has happened to you—that there were times when someone got too close to you in a way you didn't like.*

Ronald: *Yes...I didn't like it when one of my uncles tickled me. He wouldn't stop.*

Therapist: *Yes, and you didn't like it. When you said "enough" the other person should have listened. Rex is like you. He didn't feel you listened, so he asked me to tell you. We are talking about something specific. It is called "victim empathy." What that means is that if you remember your own feelings when you didn't like what was happening to you or when you wanted to be left alone, then you will be able to understand how another person or animal is feeling. Because you know how it feels, then you will be able to respect their feelings, like you want people to respect yours. That is "empathy," an important skill for all of us to learn.*

Ronald: *Why does Rex feel like that? He usually likes what I do.*

Therapist: *Animals are like people. How they feel about something may vary from day to day. Maybe Rex didn't get enough sleep last night. Or maybe Rex has an upset stomach or sore muscles.*

On these occasions, Ronald would back off for a few moments and then try to resume the unwanted behavior. The therapist would intervene, saying, "Look at the way Rex is responding to you. I don't think he is ready yet." There were times when Ronald would persist with the unwanted behavior and she would say, "Unless you can respect Rex and his needs, I won't be able to bring him in here. Having Rex here is a privilege you earn." The therapist's warnings taught Ronald the important lesson that the responsible adult in a situation would keep everybody safe, and Ronald ceased treating Rex aggressively.

AniCare Child emphasizes the significant role that animals can play, both in children's development and in clinical interventions. To involve animals in the therapeutic process does not necessarily require using an animal like Rex as an assistant therapist or even using puppets. In his work with children who have abused animals, Richard Ruth, a psychoanalytically oriented clinician, involves the entire family when working with the abused animal. He speaks directly to parents about the need to ensure the well-being of the animal. (He only does this if he first determines that the parents are functioning effectively.) He explains that it is not only important in ethical terms but that ensuring the animal's safety is important to the child's recovery. The child needs to see his parents acting in that parental capacity. After an episode of abuse, Ruth has found that families can learn about care through the process of parents and child coming together to think about and care for an animal.

In addition, all therapists can engage in empathy-building exercises and interactions. Some will occur spontaneously in the therapy. However, it is recommended that therapists deliberately and methodically teach empathy to children who abuse animals. Responding empathetically, especially based on a sympathetic concern to help the other, and committing acts of cruelty are not compatible. In this way, increasing children's capacity for empathy is one approach to reducing juvenile animal abuse.

"Empathy Skills" (DVD, Treatment submenu) reviews relevant empathy exercises and illustrates a projective technique, Interactive Drawing Technique, that is useful in empathy training (case featuring Joel).

4.3   Self-management

Cognitive behavioral therapies focus on concrete steps the child can use for changing and improving his or her behavior, emphasizing the connection between thoughts and behavior. Self-management and parent management skills are emphasized by a number of cognitive behavioral approaches, some of which have promising outcomes, according to research. For example, Carolyn Webster-Stratton and her colleagues at the University of Washington have a comprehensive program for the treatment of antisocial children, their parents, and teachers. In an evaluation study of 97 children ages 4–8 and their families, the most effective treatment was a combination of child and parent training. We address strategies of parent training below (Sect. 4.4, pp. 89–100). Children showed significant improvements in problem-solving and conflict management, and these gains were maintained in a one-year follow-up study. Unfortunately, behavior problems at school did not improve, demonstrating the setting specificity and instability of conduct problems at a young age (Webster-Stratton & Hammond, 1997).

Self-management skills are closely associated with cognitive behavioral therapies; however, other theoretical orientations also employ this method. For example, Fonagy and Target (1996) describe the goals of a psychodynamic approach as helping the child identify what thoughts make them feel things, as well as what they say to themselves.

AniCare Child presents four examples of self-management skills:
- Problem-Solving Steps
- Anger management exercises
- Self-Awareness and Stop and Think approaches
- "Animals-at-Risk" TAT

4.3.1   Problem-Solving

A cornerstone of working with children who demonstrate behavioral problems is to teach them problem-solving strategies to manage their behavior. Many problem-solving strategies are availability for use with children. The basic components of a problem-solving strategy are as follows: (1) define the problem, (2) generate alternative solutions, (3) consider the consequences of each solution, and (4) evaluate the effectiveness of the solution.

One well-known and researched behavioral intervention program, developed by Kazdin and his colleagues at Yale University, includes Parent Management Training (PMT) and Problem-Solving Skills Training (PSST) for the child (Kazdin, 1996; Kazdin, Bass, Siegel, & Thomas, 1989; Kazdin, Siegel, & Bass, 1992). A recent study found improvements for the child, parent, and family's functioning over the course of treatments, with the greatest effects realized by the child. The effects also were demonstrated across child and parent symptoms, family relations, functioning, and support (Christophersen & Mortweet, 2001). Kazdin's approach includes a five-step problem-solving skills process for the child.

4.3.2   The Problem-Solving Steps and Self-statements[3]

1. **What am I supposed to do?**
   The child identifies and defines the problem.
2. **I have to look at all my possibilities.**
   The child specifies alternative solutions to the problem.
3. **I had better concentration and focus.**
   The child evaluates the solutions that she or he has generated.
4. **I need to make a choice.**
   The child chooses the answer that she thinks is correct.
5. **I did a good job or Oh, I made a mistake.**
   This final step asks the child to evaluate the solution: whether it was the best among those available, whether the problem-solving process was followed correctly, or whether a mistake or less-than-desirable solution was selected (in which case the process should begin anew.)

Note: These steps are used by the child to develop an approach toward responding to interpersonal situations. The steps, as presented here, provide the initial set of statements. Over the course of treatment, use of the steps changes in separate ways; for example, steps two and three merge to form a separate question ("What could I do and what would happen?"), which is then answered as the child generates multiple ways of responding and the likely consequences of each. Also, the step moves from overt (aloud) to covert (silent, internal) statements.

A variation of the Kazdin approach uses an acronym—SOLVE. Using an acronym like SOLVE that conveys the purpose of the activity can help children remember the steps and facilitate their ability to use this problem-solving strategy independently (Gray, 1990).

There are five steps to SOLVE (chart on p. 46 for use with client). Each step has three examples. Present the child with the steps, analyzing the three examples in

---

[3] From: Kazdin (1996, p. 383). Copyright © 1996 by the American Psychological Association. Reprinted with permission.

each step. Next, have the child identify problems from his or her life, particularly those involving interactions with animals and with people. Use SOLVE on those problems.

4.3.3 Applying SOLVE to Human-Animal Interactions

Select the problem (identify): *Example 1:* My dog doesn't do what I want him to do. *Example 2:* My friends want me to go with them to steal a cat and have some fun with it. *Example 3:* When I'm bored I like to tease animals.

Options (explore through brainstorming): *Example 1:* I can just ignore it. I can use a friendly voice when I talk to my dog. I can offer my dog a treat. I can go with my dog to a dog obedience school. *Example 2:* I can tell my friends I am not interested. I can try to talk my friends out of it. I can tell an adult that my friends are thinking of doing this. I can go and try to make sure that they don't get a cat. *Example 3:* When I'm bored, I can go outside and either walk or run. I can look for some friends to play with. I can write about being bored. I can listen to some music. I can play with my toys or try drawing or painting.

List (discuss pros/cons and ways to solve problem): *Example 1:* If I ignore my dog, I will still feel annoyed. I can try to use a friendly voice but sometimes that is hard when I'm mad. If I offer my dog a treat, I think he will come to me but I don't know what happens then. If I go with my dog to an obedience class, my dog will listen to me better, but I'm not sure where to find an obedience class. *Example 2:* If I tell my friends I'm not interested in stealing a cat, they might get mad at me but I will stay out of trouble. If I try to talk my friends out of it they might listen to me, but they probably won't. If I tell an adult, like my teacher, they can make my friends stop, but I don't know if my friends will get mad at me. If I go and try to make sure it doesn't happen, I might not be successful and I will get in trouble. *Example 3:* If I go outside and run around I might feel better, but maybe I won't want to do that if it is too cold or raining. If I could find some friends to play with, I would feel better if they were around. I never thought of writing about being bored. I don't know how that would work, but maybe I could try it. If I listen to some music I liked, maybe I would feel better. Playing with my toys or drawing is OK, but sometimes I get bored with my toys too, and I'm not sure I know how to draw very well.

Verify (decide which options to try): *Example 1:* I think going to an obedience school is the best solution. My dog would learn a lot and I would too. I know a store that sells pet supplies in my neighborhood; they might tell me where to find obedience classes. And I can call the humane society about classes. They probably would know. *Example 2:* The best solution is to tell an adult, like a teacher, or my counselor, or my parents about my friends. If I try to stop them, it won't work. And if an adult knows about it, maybe they can stop them from doing it again so I won't have this problem and no cats or other animals get hurt. If I do something to help an animal, I think I will feel good about myself. *Example 3*: I am going to try running when I feel bored. I want to be stronger and faster and do better at sports. I think running will help me get in better shape. And if it is raining or cold, I'll just wear something that helps me keep dry and warm.

Evaluate outcomes: *Example 1:* My dog and I learned a lot and I like my dog better now. It might be a good idea to show my brothers and sisters how to treat a dog. It would help them and I would remember what I learned in class. I might be able to take what I learned in dog obedience class and use it in other situations with the kids in school and my friends. The most important thing I remember is that you can get more out of someone if you are positive and remember that they want to feel good, too. *Example 2:* I told my counselor at school and she called the boys and their parents into school and talked to them. Those boys stopped talking to me, but I don't care because I have many other friends who don't try to get me in trouble. What I learned is that when another person or an animal is in danger of getting hurt, it is important to go to an adult so they can stop it. *Example 3:* Sometimes it is hard to run when I am feeling bored, but when I do I feel good. I think I am getting in better shape. I can run for a long time without getting tired. When I have a hard time getting myself to run I remind myself how good I feel afterwards. When I'm bored at school I can't just get up and run. But I try to remember that if I don't get in trouble, I will be able to run in gym class and at lunch time and sometimes that helps.

Note that "defining the problem," the first step in problem-solving, evolves as the child learns, through therapist guidance, to recognize as a problem more general interpersonal and psychological issues. For example, the client moves from "I did not get what I wanted" to "How can I deal better with the frustrations of everyday life?" Problem-solving, then, can become characteristic of the general work of the therapy as the client learns to frame his or her experience in terms of problems to bring into the therapy.

> "Self-management Skills Problem-solving" (Demonstration DVD, Treatment submenu) illustrates the use of the SOLVE technique, with Michael.

4.3.4 Accountability and Management of Anger and Other Feelings

Other self-management skills include helping the child control his or her anger. To that end, there are a number of exercises the therapist can use. Two examples of anger management exercises follow:

"The Most Important Things to Remember About Getting Mad Worksheet" and "Who Controls Me?" These exercises are designed to help the child identify angry feelings and situations that trigger them. The exercises also help the child take responsibility and channel negative feelings constructively.

Taking responsibility or being accountable often occurs in the context of anger management but can occur independently. In either case, it is an important issue that should be dealt with in the therapy when it does occur. Failure to accept responsibility, particularly for behaviors related to animal abuse, can block progress in the therapy. Its persistent presentation is more likely in older juveniles. To supplement the exercises in *AniCare Child* (see particularly Exercise 3 below, "They Made Me

Do It"), the adult version of *AniCare* provides a theoretical explanation and practical exercises for understanding and dealing with lack of accountability that are often useful in working with juveniles (Jory & Randour, 1999, pp, 5, 15, 17).

"Empathy Skills" (Demonstration DVD, Treatment submenu) illustrates how lack of accountability can function as a resistance to therapy (case featuring Joel).

SOLVE Strategy
Select the problem (identify):
What is the problem or situation?
Options (explore through brainstorming):
What can I do? What are my choices?
List (discuss pros/cons and ways to solve problem):
What will happen if? What can I expect?
Verify (decide which options to try):
What will happen if? What can I expect?
Evaluate outcomes:
What is the best solution?

Exercises
In order to develop anger management skills, children need to learn cognitive reframing. The list below supplies a number of positive statements that the child can use to replace negative statements that the child has learned and internalized. This list can be used as a reference throughout the course of therapy.

The Most Important Things to Remember About Getting Mad Worksheet[4]

I am in charge of my own feelings. I own my feelings. I feel them and name them. It is OK to feel angry. I learn how to express my anger in ways that are helpful. Anger is part of being a human being and that is a wonderful thing to be.

The more I learn about taking care of my anger, the more powerful I become. I don't try to control my anger; I control what I do with my anger. I gain control over how I let my anger out. I watch my thoughts. Hot thoughts keep me angry. Cool thoughts calm me down. I practice cooling off. I learn to chill myself out.

I remember that people and animals are precious and deserve our respect. I stop hurting others or myself with my anger. I watch my thoughts.

---

[4] Adapted from Lynne Namka, I Stop My Bully Behavior Kit (www.angriesout.com/catalog/p6.html/).

I watch my words. I watch my actions. I own the hurtful words and actions that I do to others. I learn about things I do when I am stressed and threatened. I stop hurting animals and people with my words and actions.

I stop blaming others and myself. Blaming does not solve the problem. Blaming someone else only keeps me upset and angry. Blaming others is a way of not respecting them. Blaming myself is a way of not respecting myself. I tell my feelings and then try to work things out.

I choose to feel good about myself through speaking out. I express angry feelings in ways that are fair to people and animals and to myself. I use my firm and fair words: "I feel_____ when you _____." I understand that animals are not trying to make me angry. I am making me angry.

I don't have to hold on to my anger. I find ways to let my anger go. I talk about my hurt feelings and angry feelings. I problem-solve something that makes me upset. I keep looking until I find someone safe to talk to about my anger. I talk about my words and actions that hurt people and animals.

I take my power! I stand up for myself. I stand up for others who are being hurt, whether they are people or animals. I learn to break into my mean thoughts that I use to beat myself up.

I feel good about learning about myself.

I am powerful when I use my fair and firm words.

Who Controls Me?[5]

Introduce the idea that it is too easy to blame others for something we do and how important it is to take responsibility for what we do. Ask the child if he or she can think of situations in which someone he knows is blaming others, rather than taking responsibility. Read the vignette below and discuss it.

They Made Me Do It!

It was a warm, quiet Saturday afternoon. Lee was sitting on the steps of his apartment building. He felt bored and alone. "I wonder where everyone is," he said to himself. Suddenly Bobby and Josie came around the corner.

"What 'ya doing, Lee?" asked Bobby.

"Nothing," moaned Lee. "I'm so bored. Got any ideas?"

"Let's go down by the school and see what's happening," said Josie.

They went to the school, but there was no one around.

"Let's break into the school and get rid of those stupid gerbils they are keeping in there," Bobby suggested.

Lee hesitated. He wasn't sure that was what he wanted to do. "I don't know." He said. "We might get caught and then we'll really be in trouble."

"No, we won't get caught," Josie said confidently. "Besides, they won't even know what happened."

"Okay," said Lee. He didn't really like the idea, but he wanted to be with his friends.

---

[5] Adapted from Schmidt, F. & Friedman, A. (1985).

They broke into Miss Jones's classroom and began grabbing the gerbils and dropping them in a grocery bag. While they were doing this, the custodian caught Lee, Bobby, and Josie and called the police. Their parents were called and told to pick them up at the police station. When Lee's parents asked him why he did it, Lee said, "They made me do it."

Discussion Questions:

1. *Do you agree with Lee? Can someone else make you do something you think is wrong?*
2. *Why were their actions wrong?*
3. *How do you think Miss Jones and her class will feel when they discover the gerbils had been hurt?*
4. *How do you think Lee, Bobby, and Josie should "make right" the wrong they have done?*
5. *What does it mean to "take responsibility" for your behavior?*
6. *Have you ever stood up against your friends for something you believed was right? Tell me about it.*

Making Feelings Work for You

The therapist can use the following exercises with a child who is having difficulty with a particular feeling, or it can be used as a general way to educate a child on how to process feelings.

- Some feelings are pleasant to experience, such as our pleasure when we win a game, eat something we like, or when we know an answer to a teacher's question. Can you name two pleasant feelings you have had in the last week? Tell me about them.
- Some feelings are unpleasant and may be difficult to feel or to acknowledge. For example, feeling ashamed, or really, really angry, or very lonely are emotions that can seem unpleasant. Can you identify an unpleasant or negative feeling that you felt recently?
- One of the most important things to remember about feelings is this: Feelings give us important information about ourselves. They let us know what we like and don't like and when something is bothering us. If we pay attention to our feelings, we can learn to use them to make things better for ourselves and to help us solve our problems. In other words, you can make feelings work for you even when they are unpleasant feelings. How do you make feelings work for you? When you notice a feeling that may be bothering you or getting you in trouble, ask yourself the following three questions:
  - WHAT am I feeling?
  - WHO is responsible for my feeling?
  - HOW can I use this feeling to help me?

EXAMPLE: Arnie is teased on the way home from school because he is younger than the other kids. He is so angry when he gets home that he sometimes throws his books at his dog or kicks her. Consider what Arnie could do to make his feelings work for him.

- WHAT am I feeling?
  "I feel really mad when those brats make fun of me. They don't know what they're talking about, but they are always messing with me."
- WHO is responsible for my angry feeling?
  "Those stupid kids want to see me get upset, but I guess they can't really make me angry. Nobody can really control me in that way. What's inside of me I decide, not anybody else. So I guess I am the one responsible for being angry."
- HOW can I use this feeling to help me?
  "Well, if I don't let myself get angry and hurt my dog that would help me. I know that is wrong. If I pay attention to my anger, I can see that I have a problem with these kids that I might need help with. Maybe I could talk to my parents. Or I could talk to the school counselor or teacher and they could do something. Or I could just ignore those kids when they tease me and don't let them get to me. I could even be friendly to them so they don't think that they have gotten to me."

4.3.5 Self-awareness and "Stop and Think"

The clinical case example below illustrates the use of the self-management skills of self-awareness and "stop and think" with a child who has abused an animal. The therapist treated a 13-year-old boy, Toby, who had been referred to her by his attorney after being charged with animal abuse. As in the previous case example, this therapist uses techniques that combine cognitive therapy with a psychodynamic approach.

Clinical Case: Toby

Background

Toby and three other boys live in a rural area in a Midwestern state. As they were walking home from school, they witnessed a squirrel run in front of another boy's bicycle. The boy was unable to avoid the squirrel and hit the animal. The three other boys claimed that Toby broke the injured squirrel's neck, eviscerated the animal, then held up the squirrel in the air, declaring, "I behold the blood of the sinners" and "Death to all Jehovah's Witnesses." After doing this, the boys reported that Toby scattered the various parts of the squirrel in the surrounding wooded area, hiding the remains. One of the boys, who was horrified, ran home to tell his mother about the incident. The mother confronted Toby, who told her he only had broken the squirrel's neck to end his suffering. He explained that his mother, a medical professional, taught him that was the correct procedure to end the life of an injured animal.

Other neighbors also heard about the incident and reported it to the police, who charged Toby with animal abuse.

Toby denied that he had tortured and mutilated the squirrel.

Toby entered weekly, reduced-fee treatment, which lasted for nine months. His mother attended the last 10–15 minutes of each of his 60-minutes sessions.

Family History/Situation

Toby's biological father and his mother divorced when Toby was 6 years old. Toby's father had physically abused him since he was an infant. The father also assaulted his wife and reportedly abused animals. His mother relocated to another state because she feared for their safety, and Toby had no contact with his biological father.

His mother stated that his great-aunt, who allegedly abused numerous members of the mother's family, may have sexually abused Toby. After his parents divorced, his mother remarried and had a second child, who suffers from a rare disease and is developmentally disabled.

Toby's mother worked an evening shift and Toby had the sole responsibility for caring for his disabled sister when his mother was not home. It was difficult for Toby to participate in after-school activities, since he needed to go home to care for his sibling so that his mother could leave for work. The therapist suggested to the mother that she look into receiving assistance for her daughter, but she refused. The stepfather, who is described as "working all the time," did not have any responsibility for caring for his child. He also did not attend any of Toby's therapy sessions.

Previous Treatment

The public school system assessed Toby when he was 8 years old because of poor academic performance and talking back to his teachers. He had trouble attending during the evaluation. (The school's assessment occurred during the same period in which Toby was being abused by his father, which was unreported at the time.)

The results of the evaluation indicated that Toby possessed an IQ in the superior range and that he did not have a learning disability. Socio-emotional testing indicated that he had conduct difficulties with mild attention problems. A neuropsychological screening found no indications of impairment. Projective testing suggested a preoccupation with fantasies of violence and little remorse. Earlier, because of his conduct problems, Toby had qualified for special education services as Seriously Emotionally Disturbed (SED) and received assistance in written language.

Toby had received therapy for about a year during the time of his parent's divorce. The primary issue during that period was the loss of his father. While Toby's abuse was addressed to a limited degree, the main focus of the therapy was the effect of the divorce on Toby.

Before entering treatment, Toby was evaluated by a group under contract to the Department of Juvenile Justice to conduct evaluations. The report diagnosed Toby as paranoid schizophrenic. On reviewing the report, the therapist questioned whether or not the evaluator had the proper training or credentials to conduct the evaluation.

Assessment

Psychological testing. The therapist administered the Millon Adolescent Clinical Inventory and the Jessness Inventory to Toby. There were no indications of any Axis I diagnoses. Concern for body image, sexual feelings, and peer insecurity were elevated scales. His scores indicated attitudinal immaturity and an elevated dependency on others.

Because of his long history of problems, his therapist recommended that Toby attend a two-week day treatment program at the local hospital before entering therapy with her. The purpose of this recommendation was to put Toby in an intensive clinical situation in which he could be closely observed and become prepared for therapy. This intervention also would satisfy the courts and his mother.

Clinical interview

Toby is a baby-faced, heavy-set boy with few friends. The therapist reported that he presented with a blunted affect but maintained good eye contact and seemed willing to discuss what he had done. She referred to the police report to clarify statements that Toby made that did not coincide with the official account. Toby denied that he had eviscerated the animal before the squirrel was dead. He explained that he broke the squirrel's neck because the animal was suffering. He also denied that he held the squirrel up in the air and declared, "I behold the blood of the sinners" and "Death to all Jehovah's Witnesses."

The therapist observed that Toby was angry about his father's abuse and also resentful that he had so much responsibility for his younger, disabled sister. A child's attitudes toward animals are an essential part of the therapist's assessment. Toby's family has two pets, a dog and a cat, who are both well cared for and who have lived with the family for several years. The therapist questioned Toby about the family pets: "What things do you do with them? Do they ever do anything that makes you mad? What happens then?" To gain insight into parental attitudes, she also asks about who disciplines the family pets. Toby, who seemed to care for the animals, responded that when the cat scratched him, he understood that "Cats are like that. It doesn't mean that they want to hurt you."

Self-awareness

Self-awareness training is meant to teach a child how to reflect on his or her actions, to step back, and to take another look at a situation or event. It teaches the child that sometimes motivations are hidden and have to be inferred from the reactions that an act provoked. Focusing on motivation, perspective-taking, and the relationship between motivations and actions requires a certain level of cognitive development. In the following case, the therapist worked with Toby to help him understand his underlying motivation for killing the squirrel in front of his classmates.

The therapist came to believe that it was just as likely that Toby did not eviscerate the squirrel while he was still living. She learned that Toby craved the attention of his peers, but with poor social skills and little opportunity for informal interaction because of his responsibilities at home, his attempts to gain attention were clumsy and ineffective. Two of the three boys with Toby at the time of the incident were Jehovah's Witnesses. The therapist believed he was mocking them and hoping to shock his classmates with his statements about the "blood of sinners" and "death to Jehovah's Witnesses."

After making the assessment, the therapist confronted Toby with this possibility.

Therapist: Now that I've gotten to know you, I've been thinking about what you did to that squirrel and why you did it. You're really a smart guy. You knew it would shock your friends. And you knew it would scare them. I think that's why you did it.

Toby: I just broke the squirrel's neck because it was in trouble. I didn't say anything. I didn't say anything weird.

Therapist: Toby, let's get real here. I'm not saying it was "weird," or that it means you are weird. I don't think two other kids both came up with the same expressions on their own. I think you did say it for the reasons I stated. We can learn something from this about how you get along with other kids that might help you.

Toby: What do you mean?

Therapist: Well, first of all, I want to hear what you think of my ideas. That you were trying to get their attention, and you were trying to get it by shocking them and horrifying them. Why make comments about Jehovah's Witnesses? And about blood, which you know is an issue for that religion?

Toby: Well, maybe I did say it (laughing). But I sure got their attention.

Therapist: That's true, you did get their attention. And I think that is one of the reasons you did it. But there were consequences to getting their attention that way.

Toby: Yeah, I sure know that. I'm here and I got the police and everybody involved.

Therapist: We are going to talk more about that—about how you get attention from other kids and better ways you might be able to do that. But for right now, I want to explore more about what else was going on with you at that time.

Toby: Like what?

Therapist: Well, like what you were feeling when you saw that they were so frightened of what you did.

Toby: That they are real jerks. They're so dumb they didn't even know I was making fun of them.

Therapist: Did it make you feel superior to them then?

Toby: Yeah, I guess it did. You should have seen their faces! How could they believe I was real? Come on! Who is that stupid? I guess they are!

Therapist: You sound very contemptuous of them. At the same time, you wanted their attention. Sometimes I think you get confused and don't know what you want—to hurt them in some way or to feel that they like you, maybe even look up to you.

Toby: Yeah. I did get a kick out of ragging on them. But I know what you mean. I guess I would like to get along with them, too. You know, hang out with them and do things. They're OK sometimes.

"Stop and Think"

The therapist's use of "Stop and Think" is similar to the SOLVE approach to problem-solving noted earlier. It is a cognitive behavioral tool to help the child reject maladaptive responses and choose more productive options by first identifying thoughts and feelings and then developing alternative responses. In the example below, Toby uses this method to learn a more healthy response to his feeling of loneliness.

The therapist used self-awareness training to help Toby identify feelings that he was unaware of, but which he acted on in ways that were against his own best interests and that harmed others. Over the course of treatment, Toby was able to talk about his own suffering at the hands of his father and his feelings of loneliness that stemmed from his unrecognized abuse. He also developed insight into his maladaptive response to this loneliness, which was to seek the attention of others in ways that were ineffective and counterproductive. Toby made a spectacle of harming the squirrel to seek his friends' attention and to counteract his feeling of loneliness around them.

After Toby acquired these insights, the therapist and Toby used the "Stop and Think" approach to develop alternative responses to his feelings of loneliness.

Therapist: *So we know now that when you start feeling lonely, you can do things that don't help you deal with that feeling and even can make things worse for you. So, let's try to examine those feelings and see if we can break them down.*

Toby: *Like how?*

Therapist: *Think back to the last time you were feeling lonely. What was the first thing that happened? Did a thought cross your mind? Or did you notice yourself doing something?*

Toby: *Oh, I get it. Let's see. I remember last night after my sister finally went to bed, I started just pacing around the room...and I think I was feeling lonely.*

Therapist: *Good! So maybe when you find yourself pacing, that is an indication that a lonely feeling is starting to rise to the surface. So the idea is to do something at the beginning of those feelings before they get too strong for you to handle.*

Toby: *I don't know what to do.*

Therapist: *Let's talk about that. I want to describe something I call the "Stop and Think" approach. It is pretty simple, but it can help you gain some control over your feelings. There is a way you can learn to make your feelings work for you instead of letting them get the better of you. I know you are a good writer. You have the advantage of being very bright, so you can use your mind. And you like being on the computer. One possibility is for you to go to your computer and write about what you are feeling. Put what you are feeling into words. Sometimes that changes the feelings.*

Toby: *I'll try it. But what if it doesn't work? What do I do then?*

Therapist: *I do want you to try it. And we can talk about what happened in here. But if it really doesn't work and you find yourself really feeling bad, if you really feel you can't handle your feelings, then you can call my answering machine. You need to understand that I may not be able to get*

*back to you immediately, but I will definitely get back to you. But when
you use the "Stop and Think" approach, there is still another step to
take.*

Toby: *Like what?*

Therapist: *When you successfully use this method, it is important to give yourself
a pat on the back, to reward yourself in some way. Pick something you
really like to do and reward yourself with that. So the steps are "stop
and think" and then "self-reward."*

4.3.6 "Animals-at-Risk" TAT

This tool can be used in various ways (see discussion of projective tools in Sect. 4.2,
p. 39). The "Animals-at-Risk" Thematic Apperception Test was designed primarily
to encourage the exploration of situations in families in which there might be tension in a human-animal relationship (see Appendix C, pp. 92–99). It elicits material
on attachment, loss, separation, discipline, and conflicts over pet care.

Projectives, like the TAT, were originally developed as devices to generate material for use in psychodynamic-based assessment and treatment settings. The diag-
nostician or therapist presented a standard set of stimulus cards to the client with the
instructions:

> I am going to show you a series of pictures. For each picture, tell a story. Make sure the
> story has a beginning, a middle, and an ending. Give the thoughts and feelings of the people
> [and animals] in the story.

The series of cards was shown and an inquiry followed in which the therapist
asked for clarifications and fuller descriptions—for example, adding thoughts and
feelings of the characters or asking for an ending (adapted from Murray, 1951).

As psychodynamic approaches were augmented by behavioral and then cognitive
behavioral therapies, the projectives were adapted for problem-solving and other skills
learning. In terms of teaching self-management, the therapist can help the child frame
alternative responses to the initial story provided by the child. For example, one scene
depicts a family entering the house and encountering their dog standing near over-
turned trash on the floor. If the child's response is that the dog will be mistreated rather
than disciplined for his behavior, the therapist might probe that reaction and explore
with the child how this situation could have been different. What could the child have
done differently? What could the parents have done? If the child and parents had
responded differently, how would things have been different? If the child's family has
a dog, what could the child do to try to prevent something like this from happening?

"Self-management Skills: Projective Techniques" (Demonstration DVD,
Treatment submenu) illustrates the use of the "Animals at Risk" in the case of
Amanda. Note the relatively directive use of the tool in the context of a client
who is in a potentially volatile family situation.

Please feel free to adapt this versatile tool to your own approach and the needs of a specific case.

4.3.7 Working with Trauma-Informed Narrative

Children for whom animal abuse is an externalizing behavior intended to reduce the distress of intrusive memories of trauma may benefit from exploring and rebuilding the narrative around these events. However, note that this technique may be counter-indicated with children for whom the animal abuse is primarily motivated by cruelty or the result of modeling violent behavior—as it may reinforce acts of proactive aggression.

The narrative exploration of the abuse of an animal allows the child to explore his or her own "self-appraisal" in context (Blaustein & Kinninburgh, 2010), both as a child who has experienced abuse or trauma and then as a child who has in turn abused an animal. Have the children create a storybook of "animals I have known" in which he or she explores positive and negative interactions and attachments. From the storybook, the therapist works with the client to build a trauma narrative. Help the child to generate parts of the story that could be included and then to choose those that would be included. Finally, work with child to compose the story—how the events are included (Martin, 1998).

Capturing the story in written and/or picture form gives children multiple opportunities to rework it in ways that integrates upsetting material. Help children identify their affective and thinking state during the process by use of the exercises in the Empathy section, particularly Emotional Tracking, Emotional Choices, and Body Scan. Help children identify ways in which they have changed their thinking and behavior. The narrative can be used to help the child be accountable for the abuse—as he or she is the "author" of the story. The child can be encouraged to share the story with caregivers. Also, the story provides a vehicle for work with the caregivers (see Sect. 4.4, pp. 89–100). They can be instructed in how to parent a child who is dealing with trauma. Through exploration of the story, they can identify ways to improve both their own and their children's affect regulation and executive function in their interactions with animals.

Case Example

Brett drew pictures of himself choking a dog. In the first telling of the story, the dog "caused" the choking by making a face that reminded Brett of a growl and an earlier memory of being bitten by a dog. He was able to draw the face on the page and revisit it in therapy.

As often happens in narrative work, on reviewing, the events unfolded in a different way: "The dog made the face, but maybe I responded because I remembered my parents fighting so much." By reworking the narrative from beginning to end, Brett was able to work through experiences of responsibility and consequences and to follow the connective threads in his life—focusing on his history of witnessing domestic violence and being the object of child abuse. Brett was able to share with his mother that a trigger of his acting out with the dog was her yelling, as her voice reminded him of his powerless hiding in his room during parental arguments. The dog's face produced a strong feeling of imminent danger, which he repeatedly took out on the animal, including breaking the dog's leg.

In sessions, he was able both to process the body experiences, thereby reducing aggressive behavior, and identify ways to master future triggers in human-animal interactions that reminded him of earlier traumatic memories.

4.3.8 Children Who Witness Animal Abuse

As noted in the Assessment section, a large number of children witness animal abuse with consequences ranging from post-traumatic symptoms to increased likelihood of themselves becoming perpetrators of animal abuse. If a child witnesses animal abuse, it is important to assess the effect of this experience on him or her. Research and clinical experience with vicarious traumatization confirm that onlookers to catastrophic or violent events can suffer from a number of symptoms, including those of post-traumatic stress disorder. Depending on the severity of the effect, the child may require long-term therapy. At a minimum, the following steps should be taken:

Expression
Allow the child to express his or her feelings related to the event. Toys, puppets, drawing, painting, and writing may be helpful for many children.

Psycho-education
Help the child identify the steps that led up to the event. Discuss what alternatives might be available if a similar situation occurs again. For example, if safe, the child could speak up and try to intervene. Perhaps he or she could enlist the help of a responsible adult or authority. Inform the child that he or she can, and should, call the local police (911) or animal control agency to report animal abuse. It may be useful to discuss alternative actions in the context of teaching a child problem-solving strategies.

It is also important to provide information and education about normal symptoms and reactions that a child experiences following a traumatic event.

Depending on the situation, the therapist may remark:

- "It is normal to have those kinds of feelings after seeing something so disturbing."
- "Sometimes children are afraid to talk about what they are thinking or feeling because they think maybe it isn't normal. But it is perfectly normal. The best thing is to talk about it with someone else."
- "Even when we didn't do anything ourselves, if we saw something bad and think we could have stopped it but didn't know how, we can feel guilty afterwards. So, it's important to sort through those feelings."

Parental Support

Review with parents the steps to take when witnessing animal abuse. These steps might include reporting the abuse to the police or local animal control agency, discussing the incident with appropriate parties in the community, and attempting to provide support for the animal's safety when possible. Encourage the parents to be open to the child's desire to talk about his feelings, to give permission to talk about the incident, and to model acceptance of feelings that arise. Instruct the parents that their most important role is to be available to listen and to ensure that their child feels safe.

4.3.9   Summary

The first three subheadings of the "Treatment" section of *AniCare Child* make the following major points:
- Children who have perpetrated or witnessed animal abuse need therapeutic intervention
- Interventions use direct approaches developed to change maladaptive behavior Interventions are organized into:
- Connection—developing and using the therapeutic relationship
- Empathy—which consists of expressing (identifying and regulating) feelings, and empathy development through exercises (pp. 34–36 and 41–43, handbook), puppet play, animal-assisted therapy, and projective techniques
- Self-management skills—using techniques for problem-solving, anger management, self-awareness, and narrative rebuilding

Most of the exercises and techniques are flexible and can be used for both empathy and self-management. The segments in the Demonstration DVD on Joel (empathy skills) and Amanda (self-management skills) illustrate this versatility: The second half of the role-play with Joel shows how the Interactive Sequence Drawing technique can help child problem-solve by generating alternative responses; the first half of the role-play with Amanda illustrates how the Animals-at-Risk TAT can elicit empathy.

4.4   Working with Parents

There is clear agreement that parents play an important role in a child's treatment. At the same time, clinicians who work with families are aware that there can be numerous obstacles to parental cooperation. Many parents lack resources, are overwhelmed and overburdened, and may not have the emotional resources to examine their own behavior and make significant changes in their lives. Effective parent involvement greatly improves the child's chance of a successful outcome, and, therefore, involving parents is an important aspect of the child's treatment.

It is critical to evaluate parents or guardians to determine if they are a potential resource. In this section, we describe several approaches that develop and utilize parents to supplement individual work with a child.

However, often parents or guardians, far from a potential resource, themselves contribute to and sustain the child's behavior. Parents often are acting out their own traumatic histories or using the child to play out a dysfunctional marital relationship. In these cases, counseling the parents should precede or be concurrent with the treatment of the child. Where this is not possible, removal of the child from the family should be considered.

Research findings clearly demonstrate that parents play a significant role in the development of aggressive behaviors in juveniles (Eron, 1987; Loeber, 1990). Parent variables that make a difference include effectiveness as disciplinarians, level of warmth and positive involvement, ability to monitor children's whereabouts, tendency to be overly punitive or emotionally rejecting of children, and level of stability and organization in the home (Cavell, 2000). In addition to parental behavior, other family characteristics have been found to be fundamentally related to antisocial behavior in children. Kazdin et al. (1992) note that "Parental stress, psychopathology and social isolation, poor parental relations, and related factors affect the onset, escalation, and maintenance of antisocial behavior."

As noted earlier, not all children who abuse animals will be diagnosed with conduct disorder or determined to have generalized problems with aggression. However, the act of animal abuse by its very nature is an aggressive act, and many of the interventions used by parents of aggressive children can be applied to various degrees. Additionally, many of these interventions are useful strategies for any parent.

In working with parents whose children mistreat animals, it is advisable to instruct parents to separate the child from any pets in the family and not to allow any contact or only highly supervised contact. No new animals should be brought into the home when the child is undergoing treatment and before it is determined that the child can interact with an animal safely and positively.

There are a variety of parent treatment models; some include a multisystem approach and integrate various therapy techniques. Multisystemic Therapy (MST), a family-based system designed for chronic, violent, or substance-abusing juvenile offenders 12–17 years of age and their families, delivers services at home, in school, and in the community. MST intervention strategies include strategic family therapy, structural family therapy, behavioral parent training, and cognitive behavioral therapy. Studies indicate a high level of effectiveness; the cost of MST is $4,500 per youth (in 1998 dollars; Henggeler, Mihalic, Rone, & Timmons-Mitchell, 1998; Kazdin & Weisz, 1998).

Another comprehensive program with demonstrated effectiveness designed for at-risk youth aged 11–18 is Functional Family Therapy (FFT). Like MST, FFT integrates systems perspectives and behavioral techniques and delivers services by one- or two-person teams in a variety of contexts, at home, in clinics, at juvenile courts, and at the time of reentry from an institutional placement (Alexander et al., 1998).

More conventional contexts such as a clinic or office setting fall into two models—those that emphasize behavioral management strategies and those which focus more on relationships and family processes (Clavell, 2000). Alan Kazdin's Yale University-based Parent Management Training (PMT) is one of the better known and researched parent training programs (Kazdin, 1996; Kazdinet al., 1992). PMT refers to the following procedures (Feldman & Kazdin, 1995):

- Instructing parents in social learning principles and techniques
- Modeling and coaching of parents in sessions and practice by parents at home Procedures and interaction patterns practiced in the session are then used in the home
- Teaching parents how to define, observe, and record behavior at the beginning of treatment

Once behaviors are defined concretely, reinforcement and punishment techniques can be applied:

- Therapist-provided education on the concepts and procedures of positive reinforcement (e.g., contingent delivery of attention and praise) and negative reinforcement (e.g., time-out from reinforcement, loss of privileges, and reprimands)
- Reinforcement for prosocial and nondeviant behavior
- Parents applying new skills to relatively simple problems (e.g., compliance, completion of chores and oppositional behaviors). As parents become proficient using the initial techniques, the child's most serious problem behaviors at home and in school are addressed (e.g., fighting, poor school performance, truancy, stealing, fire setting, and animal abuse)
- Close telephone contact between therapist and parents between sessions

Numerous studies support the effectiveness of behavioral management programs. A meta-analysis of outcomes for behavioral management treatments found significantly better outcomes for children whose parents participated in parent training programs than for children whose parents did not (Serketich & Dumas, 1996). Moeller's (2001) review of outcome research on Kazdin's Parent Management Training found that PMT produced short-term gains but that its long-term effectiveness was less certain.

Additionally, PMT appears to be more effective with younger children and is less successful with families who are socially isolated and economically disadvantaged. PMT also requires extensive training for the therapist, and few programs are available for mental health professionals to acquire PMT training (Kazdin & Weisz, 1998). There are, however, a number of behavior management-oriented manuals and materials for parents and therapists available from other sources (Forehand & McMahon, 1981; Forgatch & Patterson, 1989; Sanders & Dadds, 1993).

Another often-cited behavioral training approach for parents is the comprehensive program developed by Carolyn Webster-Stratton and her colleagues at the University of Washington (Webster-Stratton, 1996; Webster-Stratton & Hammond, 1997). Evaluation of these programs, which use videotapes to model behaviors for parents, found improvements across three treatment groups: individually administered videotape modeling, group discussion plus videotape modeling, and group discussion with no modeling (Webster-Stratton, 1989).

Carolyn Webster-Stratton's program includes components for treating children, training parents, and working with teachers. Each program component specifies the individuals for whom the intervention is intended (parents, child, or teacher), the skills that are targeted, and the objectives. The University of Washington system, which is thoroughly researched and proven to be effective in many ways, has cost as a major liability.

4.4.1 Behavior-based Parent Training Tools

Behavioral techniques used with children fall into two categories: increasing prosocial behavior and decreasing antisocial behavior, which the chart below summarizes.

Behavioral Techniques Used for Treating Aggressive Youth[6]

Increasing Prosocial Behaviors

- Modeling. A "model" performs the desired response while the child observes.
- Social reinforcement. The child receives some positive social interaction (e.g., verbal praise, a hug, a pat on the back) contingent on performing the desired response.
- Activity reinforcement. The child is allowed to perform some desired activity (e.g., to play with the parent, watch television, play outside) contingent on performing the desired response.
- Shaping. The child is first reinforced for some approximation of the demand response. Once this first approximation has been learned, the child is then reinforced only for a better approximation. This procedure is repeated until the child is making the desired response.
- Token systems. The child receives some type of symbol (a "token") contingent on performing the desired response. These tokens are later traded in for some type of desired "back-up" reinforcement.

Decreasing Antisocial Behaviors

- Extinction. The reinforcement that was maintaining the undesirable response is withheld or withdrawn. In many cases, the reinforcement is adult attention and extinction consists of ignoring the undesirable response.
- Time-out from positive reinforcement ("time-out"). The child is removed from all forms of reinforcement whenever he or she performs the undesirable response. In practice, this often results in the child being removed to some quiet part of the house for a matter of minutes.
- Consequences. Something that the child values is taken away contingent on the child performing the undesirable response. Common examples of consequences are "grounding," paying fines, and loss of use of a favorite toy.

Of the variety of Parent Management Training techniques available, *AniCare Child* presents three descriptions of behavioral management techniques. *Time-out* is

---

[6] Adapted from: Moeller, T. G. (2001, pp. 299–300).

a widely used and accepted method for parents to use to help their child learn self-control. *Effective discipline with older children* provides alternatives when time-out is no longer appropriate. *Time-in* emphasizes developing positive relations between parent and child, rather than decreasing the child's unwanted behaviors.

Time-Out

The use of *time-out* is now a fairly common parenting practice and provides parents with an alternative to physical punishment and other ineffective means to address unacceptable behavior.

Time-out procedures involve removing a child from a situation in which he or she is misbehaving and giving the child an opportunity to calm down and gain control. By removing the child from the source of stimulation, a child has the opportunity to refocus energy away from the misbehavior and direct it toward more positive behavior. The success of this procedure depends upon the commitment of the parent and the temperament of the child. Children who are particularly sensitive and might feel abandoned by removal from others may not be good candidates for this approach.

- Clearly define boundaries for the child and make sure he or she understands the reason for the time-out. Never use this procedure the first time a child misbehaves, but only after the child has been warned: "If you continue to chase the cat, you will have to go on a time-out."
- Speak calmly so the child knows you are serious, but not angry. Reassure the child of your love and affection.
- Place the child in a defined location—a special chair or in his or her room. Make sure there is nothing of interest, such as toys, television, and games, and that the child is removed from the source of stimulation. The place where the child sits for the time-out can vary, depending on the situation.
- Explain that there can be no communication with anybody during the time-out. The adult who gives the time-out must maintain it and the adult must release the child, not any other person.
- When using a timer, explain, "When the sand goes through (or the bell chimes) your time-out will be over and you may get up."
- For toddlers, you may have to attend to bathroom needs first; also gently escort toddlers to their seat.
- Older children (ages 7+) who are experienced with time-outs may be told, "When you are ready to behave, you may get up."
- If the child refuses to stay seated, gently but firmly return the child to his or her seat as many times as necessary.
- If the child persists in misbehaving after the time-out, repeat the steps.
  Other things to remember about the use of time-out:
- Use sparingly; if used too often for too many behaviors, time-out can be ineffective.
- Time-out can also be used as a preventive measure: "It looks like you need to settle down. Let's go over here where it is nice and quiet so you can settle down a bit." Once the child has quieted down, tell them, "I can see you are calmer now. Are you ready to get up?"

- Time-out periods should not be long. The recommended length of time is as little as 30 seconds or less for a young child and several minutes for an older child.

Effective Discipline with Older Children

Time-out is less effective with children approaching their teen years, as being alone becomes preferred (Scott, 1997). A more effective discipline can include loss of a privilege or luxury, taking away a child's free time or use of a favorite device (video game, cell phone), retracting permission to attend a fun event, or being given a task to do. Parents often lecture, nag, reprimand, and fuss, but often do not give a consequence.

Consequences must fit the "crime" and be monitored to be effective. A time limit always should be attached to the consequence, so the child knows there is a reasonable end and does not feel hopeless.

Scott suggests that parents be calm and brief in presenting consequences. Often only one or two sentences are necessary: "Since you ____, then your consequence is ____ for ____ hours/days." Further discussion results in the child building a case about the unfairness of the ruling or in getting angry.

Time-In

Just as important as helping parents learn how to treat noncompliant behavior is to help parents encourage positive behavior. Christophersen developed a time-in procedure, defined as "frequent and consistent physical contact with the child when he or she is not engaged in inappropriate behaviors" (Christophersen & Mortweet, 2001, p. 30). Not only does time-in encourage positive behaviors, but time-out procedures tend to be more effective when children have benefited from time-ins. Here are some guidelines[7]:

- Keep physically close to your child. Maintain close physical contact with your child, especially during boring or distracting activities or any activity in which your child may misbehave. When going shopping, at dinner, watching television, in a car, or in other situations, keep your child within easy reach.
- Keep in touch with your child. Frequent and brief (1 or 2 seconds) gentle, physical contact with your child will do more to express your love than anything else you can do. Be sure to touch your child at least 50 times each day for 1 or 2 seconds. Touch him or her any time he is not doing something wrong or something that you disapprove of.
- Special play time. Spend uninterrupted play time with your child for 20 minutes, preferably 2–3 times a week. If possible, use a room where you will not be disturbed. Provide toys that facilitate pretend play, such as crayons and paper or puppets.
- Independent play. Children need to have time to themselves—time when they can play, put things into their mouths, or stare into space—without being entertained or instructed by their parents. Give children enough freedom to explore

---

[7] Adapted from Christophersen, E. R. (1990, pp. 131–132). Copyright 1990 by Edward R. Christophersen.

the environment on their own and they will learn skills they can use the rest of their lives.

- Verbal reprimands. Children can interpret adults' verbal reprimands—nagging, complaining, and pleading—as signs that their parents do not like them. Emphasize the positive; always keep in mind the old expression, "If you don't have anything nice to say, don't say anything at all."
- Nonverbal contact. Try to make most of your physical contact with children nonverbal. With young children, physical contact usually has a calming effect, whereas verbal praise, questioning, or general comments may only interrupt what your child was doing.

4.4.2 Relationship and Family Processes

Cavell (2000) has developed a relational approach, Responsive Parent Therapy (RPT), which is based on attachment theory and the work of structural family therapists such as Minuchin. Cavell stresses the importance of the therapeutic alliance between parents and therapist and offers a detailed explanation of how to build and sustain it.

Although empirical support for relational treatment is sparse and most of the studies are anecdotal or quasi-experimental, Cavell concludes that relationship-based strategies have promise.

AniCare Child follows Cavell's emphasis and proposes that the connection or therapeutic alliance between the therapist and parent is as important as it is between therapist and child. Cavell's description of the therapeutic alliance, with examples, is presented below.

Building the Therapeutic Alliance
Cavell (2000) proposes that the therapist build and maintain the therapeutic alliance through three techniques: teaching/training, processing, and supporting. Teaching and training consist of providing instruction to the parent, modeling behavior for them, and providing rehearsal and feedback.
Instruction
- Place all instruction to parents in a meaningful context; present them with the overall organizing framework for the approach
- Limit instruction to small and manageable messages
- Emphasize learning new skills rather than eliminating old ones
  Modeling
- Be careful not to intimidate parents by performing too well
- Demonstrate parenting skills in sessions with the child, using a "let's pretend" approach
- Have the parent play the part of the misbehaving child
- Encourage parents to borrow lines and approaches that other parents and adults use successfully with children
  Rehearsal and Feedback
- Focus on one skill at a time and build skills incrementally
- To reduce parents' inhibitions, keep low-key

- Make smooth transitions from rehearsal to feedback, or to additional instruction and modeling, without making parents feel that they are being graded
- "Sandwich" corrective comments between positive comments
- Provide less, rather than more
- Give clear and specific positive feedback, but provide less definitive negative feedback
- Provide constructive feedback by describing a hypothetical third party (e.g., "One mom I knew...")
- Offer coaching—feedback during rehearsal—so that parents immediately see the effect of a specific suggestion
- Provide written guidelines for conducting home rehearsal and discuss these in the session before the parents use an intervention at home

A therapist's work with Philip, a 9-year-old Caucasian boy referred to her for problems with anger management and impulse control, illustrates some teaching/training techniques.

Clinical Case: Philip

When Philip was angry or frustrated, he would engage in inappropriate and aggressive behavior. On numerous occasions, he had been overly rough with the family guinea pig.

At the initial meeting, the therapist instructed the mother to separate Philip from the guinea pig at all times until he gained control over his behavior. Philip's desire to have contact with the guinea pig and to acquire another pet became an important incentive in his treatment.

Therapist: *Philip and I will be working on anger management skills. I've talked to him about how there are always choices and consequences to those choices. We will focus on helping him make better choices to achieve more desirable consequences. You've given me a couple of examples of how he acts inappropriately when he is angry or frustrated. For example, you said that Philip would be pretty heavy-handed with the family guinea pig when in that state.*

Mother: *Yes, whenever he got frustrated by one of the other children, his father, or me, or just from playing with Tootsie much too roughly. I didn't like that.*

Therapist: *Yes, and on your own you decided to not let Philip have any contact with her. That is a very good idea. It will protect Tootsie, help Philip learn that there are boundaries, and give him an opportunity to learn how to regulate his angry feelings. As he demonstrates he can control his feelings, he can earn the privilege to spend time with her.*

Mother: *I'd go for that! How does it work?*

Therapist: *Let's talk about Philip losing control. Can you look at him and see that he may be getting ready to lose it?*

Mother: *Well, yes. Sometimes I just know that if we say "no" to something he wants, he will lose it and have a tantrum. And he also gets this look on his face.*

Therapist: *Tell me about that look.*

Mother: He starts to frown and purses up his mouth. Then he gets going and starts stomping around—and it goes on from there.

Therapist: Good; you are an observant mom. What we can do is work together to teach Philip how to control his temper. I have talked to him about learning to notice, right at the beginning, that he is about to lose his temper and to use a phrase to remind himself to stop what he is doing. The phrase is meant to stop action, and then the next step is for him to redirect that action. The catch phrase should be a word that is about something that is special to him and not something he does every day. Can you guess what Philip chose as his phrase?

Mother: Probably something to do with eating.

Therapist: You're right; it's "pizza."

Mother: That sounds like him.

Therapist: This is how you can help. You are a good observer and you notice when he is beginning to lose it. And you know the kind of situations that provoke him. So, whenever you see him begin to lose it—to have that look you described—walk up to him and softly, but firmly, say, "pizza." You don't have to do anything else and it can be a fun game between you. When Philip hears that word, either because you said it or he thought it, he knows that he is supposed to do something else—like count to 10, go into his room and listen to some music, or talk to himself.

After some period of time, Philip began to gain more control of his feelings and not react angrily when frustrated. After talking with Philip and his mother, they agreed that Philip had made significant improvements and that Philip should be allowed to have supervised contact with Tootsie, the guinea pig. After this achievement, the mother remarked that Philip had always wanted a puppy.

Mother: You know, Philip has always wanted a puppy; I know he still does.

Therapist: Yes, Philip has mentioned that to me, too. What do you think of that? Would your family be interested in a puppy at some point? Do you feel that your family is willing to take on that kind of commitment and responsibility?

Mother: Oh, yes. We all love dogs. I grew up with them, so did my husband.

Therapist: Philip is not ready yet for a puppy. However, I think earning the right to have a puppy would be a great incentive for him to continue working on his anger management skills.

The therapist spent time discussing with Philip what it would mean to take care of an animal. She emphasized the responsibilities involved and the commitment required, as well as the satisfactions gained from having an animal friend. The therapist and mother discussed ways in which the mother could reinforce this message at home. The mother thought of having Philip make a list of all of the things that he would have to do if he had a dog. She also visited the local humane society and picked up literature for Philip about pet care. After about a year of therapy, Philip demonstrated that he had reliable control over his anger and a puppy was successfully introduced into the family.

Processing with parents what they thought or felt about a certain therapeutic interaction is another important component of the therapeutic alliance. The parents of difficult children face a daunting task, and often they have a shortage of skills or a lack of support. Cavell (2000) notes they need both better skills and emotional support and suggests that the therapist move slowly between both needs.

The key to good processing is for the therapist to suspend any assumptions about why the parents do what they do or what they are going to say about what they did. To illustrate processing, Cavell (2000) offers the following example of a mother who resisted the idea of time-out and claimed that they had not worked before with her son. Cavell recommends that the therapist first learn more about the mother and acknowledge what he or she does or doesn't know about her.

> One thing I've learned about you is that you feel very strongly about the things you believe. You have let me know very clearly that you are tired of people telling you how hard it must be. And, you're tired of folks like me trotting out the same old stuff about time-outs and setting limits. So I have a pretty good idea about what you don't want. What I'm not sure about is what you do want. Can you help me there? Are you clear on what you want, or is that confusing for you, too? (p. 87)

Processing can help identify why strategies are not working, assist the parent to adapt existing strategies, and find alternatives. When parents feel that someone is really listening to them, they can more easily identify and process their emotional reactions and fully participate in the treatment.

Supporting parents entails trying to understand the parents' subjective experiences, communicating that understanding to them, being tolerant of their views and feelings, and empowering them to act on their own behalf. The therapist needs to maintain a sustained focus on the parent, which requires identifying resistance, spotting dysfunctional belief systems before getting caught up in them, and approaching parents in a way that disconfirms their pathogenic ideas about relationships.

Parents of children who abuse animals may be defensive, a common reaction of parents of aggressive or challenging children. Providing therapy to parents can be difficult and has many potential pitfalls. Overcoming resistances and repairing breaches in the therapeutic alliance, however, can be one of the most effective events in therapy.

> Cavell (2000) offers an example drawn from a case in which a resistant mother was being encouraged to engage in more positive interactions with her son. In this case, he notes that the therapist might conjecture that the mother is operating from her assumption that she will not be helped or understood by another person. Cavell asks: "Should one point out this underlying belief and suggest that it is not based in objective reality? Should one ask her to suspend temporarily her distrust and treat skills training as a type of experiment that will reveal to her the value of one's help?" He recommends a less risky tactic that may help her "break set." He remarks, "Consider for example, if this mother were told, 'You seem a bit disengaged right now. That makes me think I'm missing something—that I've not got the whole picture of what it's like for you to be this child's mother day in and day out. What am I missing? What part am I clueless about?'" (p. 82)

In the case of Philip, the mother was very cooperative with the therapist and able to learn new techniques readily. For a variety of reasons, not all parents find it easy to work with a therapist. Many parents are overwhelmed with their own needs and family demands and have difficulty acquiring and implementing new strategies for interacting with their children. In the following case, a therapist was talking to a mother and her 10-year-old son. The therapist had tried to help the mother with a number of parent management techniques, but the mother had been unsuccessful. In front of the child, the mother complained.

Mother: *He's an ugly child. He's just no good. He's so bad; he's all bad!*

Therapist: *No. He is not bad. His behavior is bad. That is an important difference to remember.*

Mother: *Sometimes I just see this nastiness and evil in him.*

Therapist: *I need to interrupt you. I know you don't intend to, but talking like that about your son is counterproductive. The words are hurtful to your son and you can't take back words.*

The mother started to cry and responded that she might have to withdraw her son from therapy. The therapist realized that she would have to give the mother more attention and spend more time with her. Typically, the therapist would talk to a parent for about 5 minutes at the end of each session with the child. After this incident, the therapist adjusted the schedule to spend more time at the end of each session with the mother. During one meeting, the therapist noted that the mother was referring to herself in negative terms, saying, "I'm just a rotten mother."

Therapist: *From what you tell me about growing up, you've accepted your parents' view of you. What you say about yourself sounds like what they said about you.*

Mother: *I'm no good. Look, I can't even raise my own son without help.*

Therapist: *I think there is another way to look at that. You are acting responsibly. You found help for your son. You come here every week. You show up on time. You are making an investment in time, energy, and money to help your son. I see you cry, which means to me that you really do care. You are replaying tapes with your son that your parents put in your head.*

Mother: *I guess I do sound like that sometimes.*

Therapist: *How did it feel for you when you were a child and they said you were no good?*

Mother: *I didn't like it. It hurt me. And it made me angry.*

Therapist: *Of course. What we are learning is that you don't have to keep on playing those tapes.*

In summary, Sect. 4.4 presented a variety of approaches and techniques. *AniCare Child* describes the general methods of a behavioral management approach to parent training, providing specific steps for three techniques, time-out, effective discipline with older children, and time-in. In addition to these behavioral management-oriented approaches, *AniCare Child* discusses the importance of the therapeutic relationship between therapist and parent and offers examples of how to build and maintain that connection.

Appendices

5.1   Appendix A

Animal-Related Experiences

10 Screening Questions for Children, Adolescents, and Adults*

1. Have you or your family ever had any pets? ....Y_____ N_____

How many?

a. Dog(s) _____   f. Turtles, snakes, lizards, insects, etc. _____

b. Cat(s) _____   g. Rabbits, hamsters, mice, guinea pigs, gerbils _____

c. Bird(s) _____   h. Wild animals (describe) _____

d. Fish _____   i. Other (describe) _____

e. Horse(s) _____

2. Do you have a pet or pets now? ....Y_____ N_____

How many?

a. Dog(s) _____   f. Turtles, snakes, lizards, insects, etc. _____

b. Cat(s) _____   g. Rabbits, hamsters, mice, guinea pigs, gerbils _____

c. Bird(s) _____   h. Wild animals (describe) _____

d. Fish _____   i. Other (describe) _____

e. Horse(s) _____

3. Did you ever have a favorite or special pet? ....Y_____ N_____

What kind? _____

Why was that pet special? _____

4. Has a pet ever been a source of comfort or support to you – even if you did not own the pet (e.g. When you were sad or scared?)..Y_____ N_____

K. Shapiro et al., *The Assessment and Treatment of Children Who Abuse Animals*,
DOI 10.1007/978-3-319-01089-2_5, © Springer International Publishing Switzerland 2014

How old were you?

_____ a. Under age 6   _____ b. 6-12 years   _____ c. Teenager   _____ d. Adult

Describe the pet and what happened _____

_____

_____

5. Has your pet ever been hurt?...Y_____ N _____

What happened? (describe) _____

_____

_____ a. Accidental? (hit by car, attacked by another animal, fell, ate something, etc.)

_____ b. Deliberate? (kicked, punched, thrown, not fed, etc.)

6. Have you ever felt afraid for your pet or worried about bad things happening to your pet?...Y_____ N _____

(describe)_____

_____

_____

Are you worried now? .... Y _____ N _____

7. Have you ever lost a pet you really cared about? (e.g. Was given away, ran away, died or was somehow killed?) ....Y _____ N _____

What kind of pet? _____   If your pet died, was the death:

_____ a. Natural (old age, illness, euthanized)   _____ b. Accidental (hit by car)

_____c. Deliberate (strangled, drowned)   _____d. Cruel or violent (e.g. pet was tortured)

What happened? _____

_____

_____

Was the death or loss used to punish you or make you do something? ....Y _____   N _____

How difficult was the loss for you?

_____ a. Not difficult   _____ b. Somewhat difficult   _____ c. Very difficult

How much does it bother you now?

_____ a. Not at all   _____ b. Somewhat   _____ c. A lot

How did people react/what did they tell you after you lost your pet?

_____ a. Supportive   _____ b. Said it was your fault   _____ c. Punished you   _____ d. Other _____

How old were you?

_____ a. Under age 6   _____ b. 6-12 years   _____ c. Teenager   _____ d. Adult

8. Have you ever <u>seen</u> someone hurt an animal or pet? ....Y _____   N _____

How many?

a. Dog(s) _____   f. Turtles, snakes, lizards, insects, etc. _____

b. Cat(s) _____   g. Rabbits, hamsters, mice, guinea pigs, gerbils _____

c. Bird(s) _____   h. Wild animals (describe) _____

d. Fish _____   i. Other (describe) _____

e. Horse(s) _____

What did they do?

_____ a. Drowned   _____ g. Burned

_____ b. Hit, beat, kicked   _____ h. Starved or neglected

_____ c. Stoned   _____ i. Trapped

_____ d. Shot (BB gun, bow & arrow) _____ j. Had sex with the animal

_____ e. Strangled   _____ k. Other (describe) _____

_____ f. Stabbed

Was it _____ a. Accidental? _____ b. Deliberate? _____ c. Coerced?

How old were you? (mark all that apply)

_____ a. Under age 6 _____ b. 6-12 years _____ c. Teenager _____ d. Adult

Were they hunting the animal for food or sport? ....Y _____ N _____

Did anyone know they did this? ....Y _____ N _____

What happened afterwards? _____

_____

_____

9. Have you ever hurt an animal or pet? ....Y _____ N _____

How many?

a. Dog(s) _____   f. Turtles, snakes, lizards, insects, etc. _____

b. Cat(s) _____   g. Rabbits, hamsters, mice, guinea pigs, gerbils _____

c. Bird(s) _____   h. Wild animals (describe) _____

d. Fish _____   i. Other (describe) _____

e. Horse(s) _____

What did you do?

_____ a. Drowned   _____ g. Burned

_____ b. Hit, beat, kicked   _____ h. Starved or neglected

_____ c. Stoned   _____ i. Trapped

_____ d. Shot (BB gun, bow & arrow) _____ j. Had sex with the animal

_____ e. Strangled   _____ k. Other (describe) _____

_____ f. Stabbed

Was it _____ a. Accidental? _____ b. Deliberate? _____ c. Coerced?

How old were you? (mark all that apply)

_____ a. Under age 6   _____ b. 6-12 years   _____ c. Teenager   _____ d. Adult

Were you hunting the animal for food or sport? ....Y _____   N _____

Were you alone when you did this? ....Y _____   N _____

Did anyone know you did this? ....Y _____   N _____

What happened afterwards? _____

_____

10. Have you ever been frightened—really scared or hurt by an animal or pet?   ....Y _____   N _____

What happened? _____

Are you still afraid of this kind of animal or other animals?..Y _____   N _____

(Describe) _____

Demographics

Date: _____

Current grade or highest grade completed: _____

Date of birth: _____ Age: _____
                                                               (years)   (months)

Gender: Male _____   Female _____

Ethnic Group: Caucasian _____   Asian _____   African-American _____   Hispanic _____

Native-American _____   Appalachian _____   Other _____

Maternal level of education (highest grade completed) _____

*Adapted from Boat (1999)

5.2   Appendix B

Psych/Social History*

Name: _____   Today's Date: _____

Family of Origin History

How many brothers and sisters do you have and where are you in the birth order? _____

To whom in your family do you feel closest? _____

Were your parents separated or divorced?_____ How old were you? _____

With whom did you live with when you were growing up? _____

How did your parents get along with each other? _____

Did you have a relationship with both parents? _____

Describe your family and childhood. _____

Has anyone physically or emotionally abused you?_____ Who? _____

Did anyone in your family have a problem with drugs?_____ Alcohol? _____

Circle which person (s):   Dad   Mom   brothers/sisters   aunts/uncles   grandparents

Do your parents or grandparents have mental health problems? _____

If so, what kind? _____

As a child, did you have companion animals?_____

If so, what happened to them?_____

How often did you move? _____ Have you been neglected or abandoned by your parents? _____

Has anyone close to you died?   _____Yes   _____No

Relationship of that person to you: _____ Cause of death:_____

Were either of your parents in the military? _____

Relationship History

Are you currently involved in a relationship? _____Yes _____No

If yes, how long? _____

Describe your partner _____

Describe your partner's attitude toward you _____

How do you feel about your partner? _____

Have you ever thought your partner was cheating? _____

Have you ever followed your partner or "checked up on the partner" to see what he/she was doing? _____

Do you think that you are jealous or possessive? _____

How many serious relationships have you had? _____

Have you had an affair or cheated on someone? _____

How long was the longest relationship that you have had? _____

Have you ever been divorced or separated? _____How many times? _____

Do you prefer sexual relationships with _____women? _____men? _____both?

List your children and stepchildren. Put a check mark next to those not currently living with you.

Name	Age	Name	Age

Education and Employment History

What was the highest grade you completed in school? _____

Did you graduate from high school? _____What year? _____

If no, do you have a GED? _____

Did you have learning difficulties in school?_____

If yes, briefly explain? _____

Did you ever get into trouble in school? _____

If yes, what happened? _____

Were you ever expelled or suspended from school?_____If yes, for what? _____

Did you ever have problems with teachers or neighbors? _____

If yes, what happened?_____

What is your current employment?_____

How many jobs have you had in the past 5 years?_____Have you ever had a problem with a boss?_____

Have you ever been fired?_____ If yes, why? _____

_____

How long have you been with your current job? _____

Legal History

How many times have you been arrested? _____Were you arrested as a juvenile?_____

Have you ever been arrested for domestic violence? _____How many times? _____

Have you ever been stopped for DWI or DUI? _____How many times? _____

Have you ever been arrested for a felony?_____

Please list the dates and reason for each arrest (regardless of conviction):

_____   _____

_____   _____

_____   _____

Do you currently have any outstanding warrants for your arrest? _____

Where? _____

Psychological History

Have you ever been in counseling or had to take classes?_____

Where? _____

For what? _____

Have you ever thought of suicide? _____ If yes, why? _____

When was the last time you thought about suicide?_____

Are you still thinking about it?_____ What was your plan? _____

What is going on in your life when these thoughts occur? _____

Have you ever had any of the following?

_____Phobias (intense fear)   _____Delusions   _____Fear of going crazy

_____Panic attacks   _____Hallucinations   _____Thoughts of killing someone

Violence Behavior Checklist and Assessment

Have you EVER done any of the following?

_____Slapped, kicked, or shoved your partner   _____Blocked partner's path

_____Slapped, kicked, or shoved children   _____ Indulged in mocking or name calling

_____Hit your partner or children   _____Withheld affection/sex

_____Punched walls or broken personal property   _____Restrained partner/person

_____Threatened to leave or divorce partner   _____Drunk or done drugs to relieve anger

_____Become more angry as a result of drinking or drugs

_____Threatened someone with a weapon   _____ Threatened family, children, or pets

_____Hurt an animal   _____ Except for hunting, killed an animal

_____Had sex with your partner when he/she didn't want to

_____Have you ever disciplined your children more than you meant to?

_____ What type of discipline do you use with your children? _____

_____ Have you ever disciplined pets more than you meant to?

_____ Have you ever been abused _____ physically? _____ sexually? _____ emotionally?

By whom? _____

Please check the experiences that you have witnessed:

_____ Parents hitting/hurting each other   _____ Parents hitting/hurting you

_____ Street crime   _____ War

Have you ever been in any fights (with friends, in bars, at school, ect.)? _____

Drugs and Alcohol Use History

What drugs have you tried? Please check:

_____ (Pot) Marijuana   _____ Cocaine or crack   _____ Downers

_____ Meth or Crystal Meth (Speed)   _____ LSD or PCP   _____ Other   _____ Inhalants

How old were you when you first drank alcohol? _____   Did drugs? _____

How often do you drink? _____   How often do you get high? _____

Have you ever gotten high on prescription drugs? _____   What drug(s)? _____

Have you ever gotten high on over-the-counter drugs? _____

When was the last time you drank or got high? _____

If we do a urine test today, will it be hot (positive)? _____

Have you ever felt you needed to cut down on your drinking or drug use? _____

If yes, briefly explain: _____

What was the longest period you have been able to remain drug/alcohol free? _____

How many times have you been to any of the following?

_____ Detox   _____ DUI classes

_____ Residential treatment   _____ Halfway House

List the programs or agencies in which you have been in treatment or classes for drug or alcohol:

Program   Name   Year

_____

_____

_____

Have you ever attended Alcoholics Anonymous or other 12 Step meetings?_____

Why? _____

How often have you had the following when you did drugs or drank?

_____Memory loss or blackout   _____Loss of control (drank or used more than you intended)

_____Personality changes   Please describe _____

_____Stealing, sneaking or lying about, or hiding drugs or alcohol

Describe the consequences you have experienced from your drug or alcohol use

Legal consequences: _____

Personal consequences: _____

Medical Survey

How would you rate your health?   poor _____   average_____   excellent _____

Are you currently under medical care? _____For what reason? _____

Are you taking any medications or prescription drugs? _____For what reason?_____

Name of your doctor: _____ Last time you saw your doctor: _____

Have you ever had any of the following? Seizures _____Heart problems _____

Learning disabilities _____ Head or brain injuries _____

FOR WOMEN: Are you pregnant?_____If yes, are you receiving pre-natal care?_____

Military

Have you ever been in the military? _____How long?_____

If yes, what kind of discharge do you have?_____

What is your veteran status? _____

Is there anything else we should know about you? _____

_____

*Adapted from an intake protocol of the Aurora Center for Treatment, Aurora, CO (unpublished).
To be filled out by parent or caretaker of child.

5.3   Appendix C

5.3.1   Use of the "Animals-at-Risk" Thematic Apperception Test[1]

Randall Lockwood

The enclosed illustrations were used during subject interviews in the course of our study of the care of pets within families with a history of child abuse, neglect, or endangerment (Deviney, Dickert, & Lockwood, 1983) and an unpublished follow-up with these families. They were primarily used as a stimulus to encourage discussion of events that might transpire within the family surrounding common situations that might create tension in the human–animal relationship. In practice, they proved to be very helpful in eliciting comments about the use of discipline, family conflicts over pet care and issues of pet loss, disposal or abandonment. One of the most revealing questions in the course of a child interview can be "What happens when a pet does something wrong?"

Although loosely based on concepts explored in the Roberts Apperception Test for Children (Roberts, 1982), these pictures do not constitute a standardized or validated assessment tool, and we did not create a quantifiable scoring system for their use. However, such illustrations have been helpful to counselors, therapists, school psychologists, and others seeking greater insights into the dynamics of pet-owning families with possible discipline or violence issues. They have been employed in both group and individual therapy.

Other studies have demonstrated that similar illustrations can quickly reveal attitudes toward animals and the influence of those attitudes on the perception of people who are associated with them (Lockwood, 1983, 1985). We have also demonstrated that attitudes and emotions revealed by such illustrations can correlate with physiological responses to the presence of companion animals (Friedmann & Lockwood, 1991).

Please feel free to make use of these items in your practice; however, they are not to be reproduced, published, or sold without my permission.

---

[1] The stimulus cards on the following pages are redrawings of the originals in Lockwood, to provide ethnic diversity and reflect more current fashion, furniture, and technology.

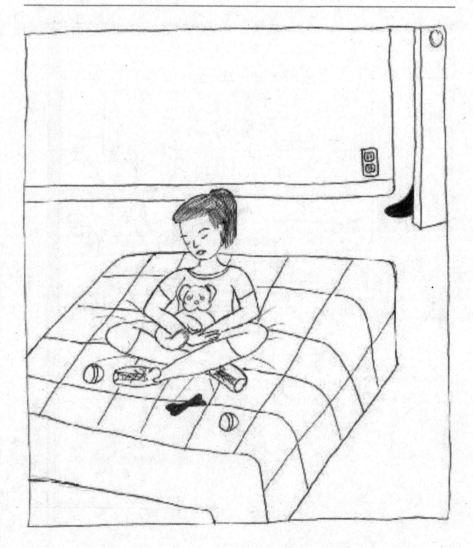

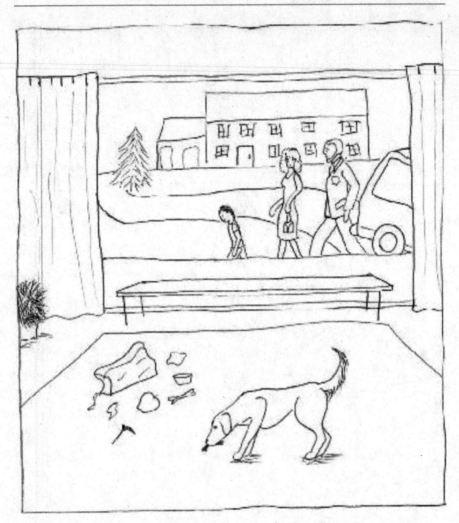

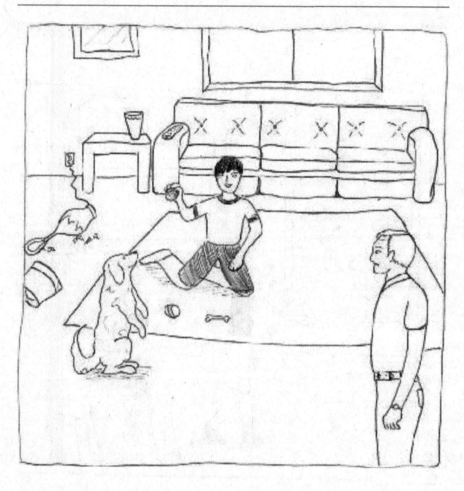

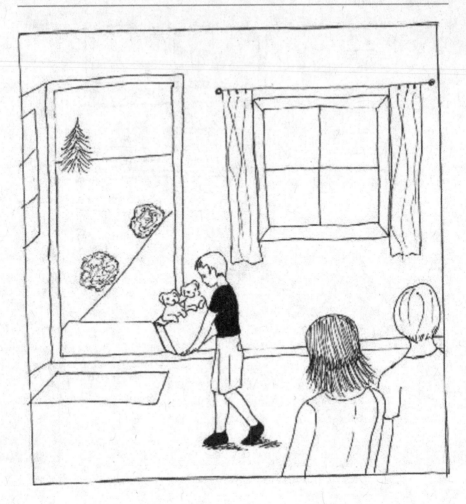

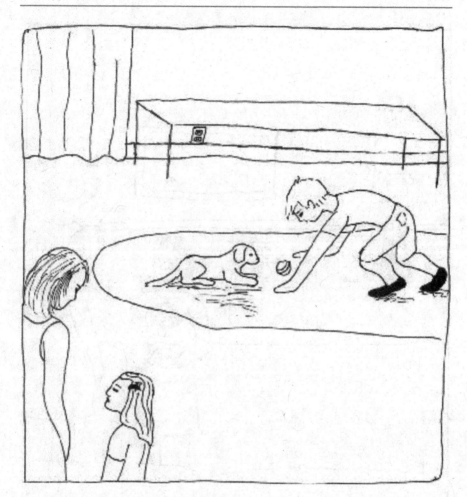

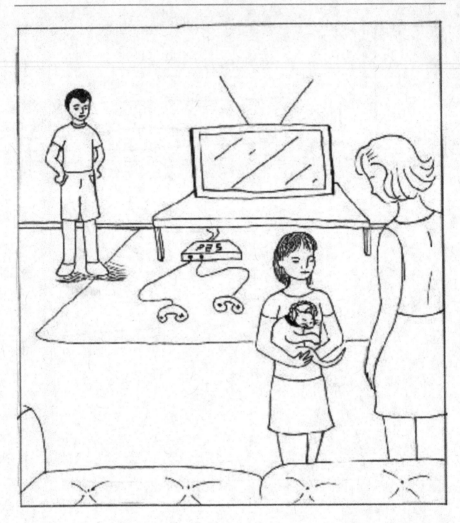

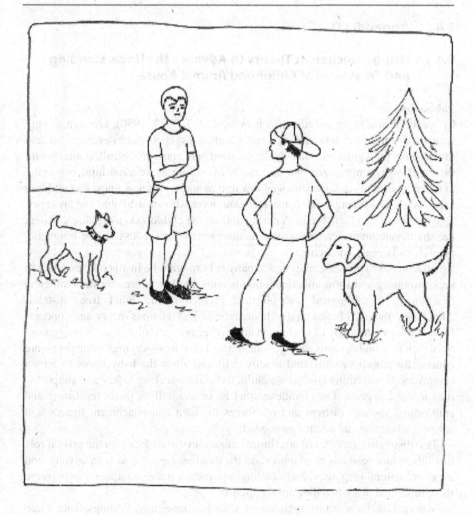

5.4   Appendix D

5.4.1   Using Attachment Theory to Advance the Understanding and Treatment of Childhood Animal Abuse

Pat Sable

Concepts of attachment, credited to Bowlby (1969, 1973, 1980), are increasingly seen as a significant approach to understanding psychological development and functioning throughout the life cycle. In what has come to be called attachment theory, Bowlby emphasized that the quality of our closest relationships, beginning in infancy, sets the stage for who we grow into as adults. We now know that children need loving attachments with consistent caregivers who are available and appropriately responsive to their needs. A caring and secure childhood environment fosters healthy development. Precarious connection, separation, or loss can be traumatic, painful, and deeply damaging.

Attachment theory describes how a baby is born with the instinctive tendency to seek proximity and form affectional bonds with familiar figures for the biological function of psychological and physical protection and relief from distress. Attachment theory is based on psychoanalytic-object relations theory and concepts from ethology (the study of nonhuman animal behavior), evolutionary biology, cognitive science, and systems theory. Attachment behaviors—crying or clinging—are genetically preprogrammed and readily activated when the baby needs to attract caregivers. If something frightens a child, the child—seeking safety and support—runs to the caregiver. The confidence that he or she will be there, reassuring and comforting, reduces distress and reinforces the idea that attachment figures will respond when they are wanted or needed.

Two distinctive features of attachment theory are (a) its focus on the pivotal role that this secure base has in adaption and (b) that feelings such as fear, anxiety, and anger are natural responses. Such feelings are part of innate equipment to preserve these relational ties when they are threatened.

Schore (2004), a neuropsychologist who has integrated findings from brain research with attachment theory, alleges that caregivers not only respond to their children's distress but also to their positive emotions such as interest and joy. This "psychobiological attunement" by the parent influences brain development in the child as well as the ability to handle feelings—such as anger—throughout the life span. Schore explains that attachment experiences are processed and stored in implicit memory in the right hemisphere of the brain, specifically in the right cortex. Once encoded in memory, these interactions endure, forming the basis of thoughts and feelings about oneself and others. When early experience is traumatic, the maturation of the developing brain is interrupted and impaired, resulting in structural limitations in a person's ability to regulate emotions.

In particular, Schore (2004) states that impairment of the right orbitofrontal area of the brain limits the ability to process and regulate negative states such as fear and aggression. The inability to regulate these kinds of strong emotions is associated with difficulty in soothing oneself, lack of empathy, and a proneness to impulsive or violent behavior. According to Schore, adolescent or adult psychopathology often can be traced to earlier relational trauma when a child's immature neurobiological system is not able either to evaluate or to regulate stress efficiently. Similarly, Siegel's (2003) work on cognitive development explains how traumatic experiences—especially continuous ones—can change human brain structures that are involved in the processing of information, thus resulting in difficulties in consolidating experiences.

Bowlby (1969, 1973, 1980) introduced the concept of internal "working models" to describe the processes involved in the continuing influence of attachment-related experiences. Working models include simple maps of the environment as well as more complicated beliefs and attitudes about oneself and others. Although somewhat automatic and relatively stable, these cognitive-affective representations are dynamic, not static. Therefore, they have the flexibility to adjust to changing conditions in either the internal or external environment.

Traumatic Attachment Experiences

Schore (2003, 2004) and Siegel (2003) are two theorists who have used findings from infant observation, cognitive and affective neurosciences, and trauma research to understand how a child's development can be diverted from resilience and competent functioning to dysfunction and vulnerability to psychological distress. Attachment-based research has identified a variety of disturbing or disruptive experiences that can compromise adaption, impairing affect regulation, cognitive flexibility, and relationships with others. These include parental threats of abandonment; withholding love; and witnessing or experiencing emotional or physical abuse, neglect, separation, or loss.

Furthermore, the effects of traumatic circumstances tend to be cumulative and also may be compounded by confusing communication from parents. Parents may prohibit events from being seen as they are, resulting in a "mismatch" between what children experience and what they are told. Because children need to retain attachment at any cost, to realize confusing communication or hostile caregiving would be too alarming or threatening. To maintain the relationships, children, therefore, may sacrifice their perceptions and comply with the demands and attitudes of others. Discordant or disorganizing attachment experiences can exacerbate emotions or cause them to be displaced. When moderate, anger often is a functional response to reproach and deters an attachment figure from repeating hurtful behavior that could endanger the bond. If protest against behaviors such as threat of separation or loss, exposure to substance abuse, or neglecting or humiliating treatment cannot be expressed, it may be misdirected to inappropriate targets (Bowlby, 1984). Calvin, who described killing a kitten because it "bothered" him, illustrates the strategy of redirecting frustration or anger rather than letting the actual source of distress be accessed.

Attachment Disorders

From a perspective of attachment, emotional distress stems from adverse attachment experiences, present and past, especially those that have compromised feelings of security and safety in relationships with others (Sable, 2000). In this vein, animal abuse might be precipitated by a form of disordered attachment behavior provoked by environmental failures such as disconfirming, abusive, or rejecting caregiving to a degree severe enough to result in causing pain and suffering to a helpless animal. One of the underlying dynamics of the behavior is a plea to repair ruptures of attachment that have gone awry. Feelings such as frustration and anger are natural when elicited to maintain attachment. When projected onto animals, however, such feelings become maladaptive, intensified, and redirected from the disappointing relationships.

It follows that if animal abuse is considered in terms of interpersonal experience, assessment and treatment must examine and understand the context in which the child lives. In support of this allegation, now there is evidence that the roots of a troubled child's behavior lie in particularly close relationships. Research also has found that parents' own attachment experiences are associated with their child's feeling of security. Whenever possible, treatment should include the parents to help them reflect on and understand how their attachment experiences may be influencing their attitudes and ability to parent their child. Encouraging parents to explore their own childhoods not only clarifies where they may have developed dysfunctional ways of relating but also shows an interest in the parents. As they come to feel safe, respected, and valued, parents will be more willing and able to participate in their child's treatment. (Techniques for assuring parents' cooperation are given in Sect. 4.4.)

Applying Attachment Theory to Treating Animal Abuse

As noted throughout this handbook, treatment must take place in a setting that feels safe to the child and the child's family. The therapist is in a position to provide an alternative kind of attachment relationship. As with any attachment, however, it takes time for a sense of security to develop. With emotional availability, a comforting presence, and continuity, the therapist gradually becomes a secure base within which to remember, reflect on, and gain a new perspective on the events and experiences that have led to the current situation.

A central feature of attachment theory is the position that maladaptive behavior stems from attachment traumas—from real experiences possibly dating back to infancy, even from parent's traumatic histories. These early traumas set up internal working models that guide relationship experiences throughout the lifespan, so that models tend to remain relatively stable over time. It is only as these relationship experiences are uncovered and affirmed that working models can begin to be changed. (The Trauma-informed Narrative exercise is a helpful tool here—pp. 53–54.) Therefore, the client is encouraged to remember and sort through memories of trauma and thwarted attachment with a goal of seeing they are the product of certain experiences that now can be reevaluated. If a child is threatened with a parent's abandonment but is afraid to express the fear and anger this could evoke, the child may let out the accompanying anger and frustration on a helpless animal. (The Animals-at-Risk TAT—pp. 52–53—can be helpful for eliciting these kinds of feelings and attitudes.)

It is through experiencing a new and safe attachment relationship, while composing a narrative of how animal abuse developed and possibly persists, that children may be able to feel differently about themselves and their behavior. Schore (2003, 2004) adds that the repetitive affective interactions that take place during therapy sessions expand right brain systems involved in coping with negative states such as aggression. He explains that accepting and affirming a client's communications—being attuned in a way that modulates emotions—restructures strategies of affect regulation and behavior.

Attachment theory makes a point of validating clients' version of their experiences while at the same time considering that they now may be seen in a new light. To question the reality of a story or to imply that a memory is imagination, fantasy, or magical thinking may make clients feel as misunderstood and discounted as they have been in other relationships. It also could raise defenses that deflect attention either from remembering traumatic experiences or from examples of what parents or other attachment figures repeatedly may have said (Bowlby, 1988; Hunter, 1991).

In addition to reexamining and reassembling events and how they are perceived, clients are helped to understand and accept their feelings, to appreciate that the alarm and anger of separation or the sadness of loss are built in, inherent responses to attain and maintain personal bonds. It can be conveyed how defensive strategies may have inhibited or intensified feelings, diminishing the ability to bounce back from adversity.

Attachment Styles

According to attachment theory, how individuals talk about themselves and their feelings reveal how they have organized their attachment experiences and how they have regulated their behavior toward others. These attachment patterns, or styles of attachment behavior, can help therapists imagine and construct a scenario of their clients' lives—including the defensive strategies the clients may have developed to deal with traumatic circumstances.

Originally, the patterns were identified simply as secure or insecure, then extended to include two insecure patterns: (a) anxious-ambivalent and (b) avoidant. These classifications were based on research findings from a structured laboratory procedure, the "Strange Situation," devised by Ainsworth, Blehar, Waters, and Wall (1978) to assess the quality of mother-child interaction. Later research by Main and Solomon (1986) added a third insecure category: disorganized/disoriented attachment.

More recently, Main and Solomon (1990) investigated adults' patterns of attachment with the "Adult Attachment Interview," a one-hour structured interview that includes questions about separation and loss experiences with parental figures. This interview has been instrumental in demonstrating an association between children's security and their parents' classification. Adults who are rated "secure" or autonomous are willing and able to speak of attachment experiences with clarity and coherence and are more likely to promote secure attachment in their children.

The patterns of insecure attachment parallel Ainsworth, Blehar, Waters, and Wall's (1978) categories of child attachment: (a) "preoccupied," which indicates over-activated attachment behavior; (b) "avoidant" or dismissing, which indicates deactivation of attachment behavior; and (c) unresolved/disorganized, which refers to individuals who exhibit a greater degree of defensive exclusion of attachment experiences. Main and Solomon argue that the incoherence of their discourse about attachment is due to early unresolved loss or trauma.

A variety of developmentally appropriate measures have been validated since Main and Solomon's initial work to determine a child's or adolescent's predominant attachment pattern (Simpson & Rholes, 1998). Although it is not possible to determine a child's attachment style without a formal administration of developmentally appropriate measure, therapists may learn much about their client by taking note of attachment-related issues such as responses to separation and loss and use of others (including animals) for support.

For example, avoidant attachment is characterized by defensive exclusion and deactivated attachment behavior. In children who abuse animals, this might be revealed in comments such as, "An animal has no emotions and does not feel pain." These children may have learned that their caregivers became annoyed or agitated in response to displays of distress; consequently, they minimize their attachment behavior and affect.

In contrast to children whose "flight from feeling" (Karen, 1994, p. 401) may cause them to downplay their attachment needs and feelings, children may show intense involvement with parents and sensitivity to separation, suggestive of an ambivalent or resistant attachment style. Ambivalent attachment is correlated with caregivers who are inconsistent and unpredictable; consequently, these children continually test their caregivers' availability by clinging and demanding attention and reassurance. Though hurt, angry, and constantly worried about the intentions and reliability of attachment figures, they allow some degree of hope that solace and affection still might be forthcoming.

The 7-year-old boy, Tony (pp. 30–33), shows elements of ambivalent attachment. Separation from his father at age 5—his mother abruptly giving away his cherished dog, combined with her inconsistent, sometimes abusive behavior—suggests that Tony felt anxious about the availability and responsiveness of attachments. His therapist recognized this apprehension, stating that Tony succumbed to his friend's destructive influence because of his need for attention and attachment.

The third pattern of insecure attachment, "disorganized/disoriented," is characterized by a greater degree of contradictory, angry, and disturbed behavior. The case of Calvin (pp. 34–37), the 9-year-old child who killed a kitten, illustrates some qualities of disorganized attachment. Children who reveal this destructiveness feel unworthy of care, perceive their parents as unavailable, and are, therefore, both fearful and angry about not having their needs met. Research has shown that the pattern persists in adolescent conduct disorders associated with unresolved and dismissing attachment (Tyrrell, Dozier, Teague, & Fallot, 1999). It is important to emphasize that experiences that could elicit these confused and frequently violent behaviors include more overwhelming mistreatments such as intrusive or neglectful caregiving, hostility, rejection, prolonged separation, or distressing loss.

Separation and Loss

Several of the illustrations in this handbook describe children who manifest an indifferent attitude toward the torment they inflict on an animal (Toby, pp. 49–52). The lack of empathy and sympathy for the pain and suffering of another suggests they have been subjected to some early relational trauma at the time in development when they were especially vulnerable to insensitive or negative treatment.

Schore (2003) notes there is flattened affect in neglected infants, which evidence suggests might be even more destructive than abuse and that this developmental trauma is linked to later hostile acting-out behavior. Schore explains that an accumulation of maltreatments, not a single event, usually causes the dysregulation of the brain's "fight" centers in the orbitofrontal cortex such as indicated by lack of empathy, together with animal abuse. Likewise, Bowlby (1973) recognized the real and serious effects of chronic stress when he began to put together a theoretical explanation of films his research assistant, James Robertson, made of young children who were separated from their parents and cared for by strange persons in strange surroundings. In trying to describe what it was like for these children to be alone, trying to cope without the comfort and support of their familiar caregivers, Bowlby identified three phases of emotional response through which the children progressed: (a) protest, (b) despair, and (c) detachment. Fear, anxiety, and anger are prominent during the first stage of protest, indicating an urgent attempt to search out and recover a missing person. The next phase of despair is a quieter, sadder time. The child is more subdued. Although still preoccupied with bringing the parent back, hope is fading: As though in mourning, the child becomes withdrawn and less active. If separation is lengthy, repeated, or harsh, the child finally moves to a defensive position of emotional detachment. This deactivation of attachment behavior is evident in reunion where the child may be unresponsive and turn away from efforts to comfort or reassure. If the rupture is not repaired or worked through, detachment can continue indefinitely, affecting the direction of developmental pathways and weakening resilience.

Separation, Anxiety, and Natural Clues

Bowlby's (1973) description of children's reactions to separation documented that the children experienced separation as a threat to their security and well-being (Kobak, 1999). Using his ethological approach, Bowlby explained that the disposition of the children to respond with fear and anxiety at the prospect of separation or loss is part of our "basic behavioral equipment" (p. 85) built into us just like fear of the dark, heights, loud noises, or strange people and things. These "natural clues" are warning signs of an increased risk of danger; we are designed to respond to them as though the peril actually exists.

The concept of separation as a "natural clue," together with the premise that it is adaptive to respond to this threat, offers clinicians a perspective for understanding and helping clients. It can be pointed out that feelings such as fear and anger are inherent responses to safeguard attachments and that certain circumstances may have intensified feelings beyond what is functional. As these experiences are clarified, it may be possible to revise and restructure working models. Some of the children cited in this manual do not feel empathy for the animal they abused. Attachment-based research has substantiated that empathy for the distress of others evolves out of being treated with empathetic and responsive care. Juvenile animal abuse suggests a failure in this development. As the therapist becomes a secure base and shows interest in understanding the client's distress and reasons for it, empathy for animals and others has the potential to develop.

Another aspect of attachment theory for treating animal abuse is Bowlby's (1988) belief that therapy should offer occasional guidance. Therapists can educate clients about animals, their behavior, and their vulnerability—that abused dogs may be suffering more than their behavior suggests because at times they do not overtly show pain. Explaining this from an evolutionary point of view, it can be speculated that it could be adaptive instinctively to act stoic and hide the pain they might feel. This reserve would protect them from attracting a predator that might see an animal who shows signs of pain or injury as easy prey (Coren, 2004).

Conclusion

From the developmental perspective of attachment theory, animal abuse represents an expression of dysfunctional anger and aggression, redirected from disturbing memories and experiences and imposed on an animal who can neither escape nor complain. As deZulueta (1993) put it: Violence is "attachment gone wrong" (p. 64). It was Bowlby's conviction that real experiences such as separation or loss, a depressed caregiver, or a tumultuous family milieu are traumatic events that can compromise development, including development of the brain. Childhood trauma is biochemically encoded into the brain, affecting the ability to regulate emotional states or process information. If the integration of cognitive and emotional processing is disturbed, the child may see the world as dangerous and unsettling, thereby being quick to lash out at a convenient target—the animal.

The therapeutic approach of attachment is to become a "trusted companion" (Bowlby, 1988, p. 138) with whom to experience a new way of being together and with whom to recover and reconsider the meaning of both current and past affectional experiences. Feeling heard and understood, feeling affirmed and valued, can enhance a child's sense of security and ability to regulate negative feelings without having to resort to animal abuse. The link that attachment data have found between childhood trauma, insecure attachment, and a propensity toward violent behavior suggests that the secure base of therapy can help children form more satisfactory relationships with both their human and nonhuman companion animals.

5.5 Appendix E

5.5.1 Supplementary Cases

Name: Andy
Age: 3
Gender: Male
Ethnicity: Caucasian

Referral: A day school teacher asked the school guidance counselor to see her 3-year-old student. The teacher reports that when she brings in animals Andy handles them roughly. For example, he poked his finger in the eye of a gerbil and slapped a visiting rabbit.

Social and educational background: Andy's parents do not report any problems with him at home. Andy's mother is expecting a second child shortly. Andy has good relationships with the other children in the preschool, although he appears to be more easily frustrated than his peers are. If he is not chosen for a group, or has to wait his turn, he often loudly protests and refuses to accept the decision.

Precipitating events: The only change or anticipated change is the birth of a sibling.

History of companion animals: There are no animals in the family. Andy's father had dogs as a child.

Self-presentation: Andy is big for his age. He immediately engages in play and is tough on the play materials.

Name: Ryan
Age: 8
Gender: Male
Race: Caucasian

Referral: Ryan is a 8-year-old foster child referred for therapy following an incident of shoving food down a dog's throat until it choked, witnessed by the foster mother and which led to his removal from the home because of concerns about his impulsivity around the many animals in the home. He also had been observed chasing several of the farm animals and squeezing them tightly. As a small toddler, Ryan had also been a witness to or actually perpetrated a squeezing of a kitten into a wooden box, which led to the animal's death. He was identified by protective services as being an abuser of animals.

Social and educational background: Ryan is currently living in a safe home, awaiting placement in a new foster home that does not have animals. Ryan had lived with his mother until his removal at the age of 6, secondary to parental neglect, substance abuse, and physical abuse. This family had a history of involvement with protective services for many years. Two of his five siblings continue to live in the foster home from which he was removed, his youngest sibling is being adopted, and he has limited contact with the older children. There is a strong family history of substance abuse and mood disorders. His father is incarcerated for a domestic violence charge. Ryan has weekly supervised visitation with his mother at the state child protective services office. He had been diagnosed with ADHD at the age of 7 and placed on medication. Secondary to the history of parental neglect and substance abuse, Ryan may meet the criteria for a reactive attachment disorder.

He is a poor student and has every indication of having a significant learning disability and reading disorder. In the two years since his removal from his mother, he has had four different foster care placements.

Precipitating events: Ryan had multiple foster care placements and had participated in an intensive outpatient program where he was diagnosed with ADHD, shortly before being seen for therapy directly related to his maltreatment of animals. Ryan reported feeling angry about the attention being paid to his siblings prior to shoving food down the dogs' throat. He also reported squeezing the farm animal tightly because he thought "it tried to steal my toy." He tended to blame and project his feelings onto the animals in the foster home reporting them as "bad," "mean," and "selfish."

History of companion animals: For the first six years of his life, Ryan grew up in a home with his mother, grandmother, and occasionally his father with multiple animals, both dogs and cats. Much of the home setting and care of animals seemed chaotic with a lack of supervision of children in their interactions with animals. Ryan remembers a "squished kitten" and "feeling sad for the dead cat." He was also bitten in the face by a family dog when he was 4. Ryan describes himself as someone who "loves animals" and "loves to chase animals." He admits to getting very excited around all animals and having difficulty keeping his body still and his hands to himself.

Self-presentation: Ryan presents as anxious, impulsive, and defended initially about the event with the dog that led to the change in placement

Name: Angelo
Age: 8
Gender: Male
Ethnicity: Hispanic

Referral: After finally catching one of two new kittens that would not come on command, Angelo sat on the kitten. Subsequently, the kitten died. Since this incident, Angelo's parents have become increasingly concerned as Angelo's behavior toward the family's small dog has become more aggressive, including kicking at her when he did not want the dog around. They referred him to counseling due to caregivers reporting of significant concerns with the safety of their home pets due to poor impulse control when engaging with and handling small animals.

Social and educational background: Angelo lives in the city with his biological grandfather and adopted grandmother, due to a history of neglect and child endangerment with his biological parents. He has two homes and time is split between grandfather and grandmother's homes. Angelo experienced both prenatal drug exposure and little to no prenatal care and has a history of frequent illness as an infant and toddler with high fevers and numerous ear infections. Angelo was diagnosed with profound hearing loss and deafness and currently wears a cochlear device. Angelo is a special education student and attends his local elementary school where is a good student, enjoying learning and friendships. He is very busy and has a difficult time concentrating. He has also been referred for OT assistance.

Precipitating events: Introduction of two new kittens into the family after the separation of grandparents and Angelo's adjustment to living in two separate households.

History of companion animals: Angelo's family currently has two small dogs. After obtaining the second dog, Angelo's behavior calmed considerably toward the new and old dog. He had two previous dogs in his short life, both older and past away from age-related issues. In addition, he had two kittens at grandfather's house. The one kitten was killed when he sat on it and the other disappeared shortly after the incident.

Self-presentation: Angelo is an energetic, outgoing young boy who is eager to participate in therapy activities and appears to be of average or above-average intelligence.

Name: Jeremy
Age: 10
Gender: Male
Ethnicity: Caucasian

Referral: His parents observed that Jeremy was irritated and sad. When they inquired, he told them about an event in which he witnessed animal abuse. He also reported that he was having trouble sleeping.

Social and educational background: Jeremy lives in an upper-middle-class suburban neighborhood. His parents are professionals. He is an only child. He is in the 4th grade, likes school, and is a very good student.

Precipitating events: One day when he was walking to a neighborhood friend's house, he heard laughing and other strange sounds he couldn't figure out. The noises seemed to be coming from someone's backyard, which was surrounded by a 6-ft-high privacy fence. Curious, he gazed through the space in the fence slats and saw two teen-aged boys and a teen-aged girl with something in their hands. Then Jeremy realized what was happening: they were restraining a cat and pouring something down the cat's throat. The cat was struggling and making strange sounds, but couldn't free himself. He heard one of the kids say, "Hey, this should really make your engine purr!" and laugh. They were forcing the cat to drink motor oil. Jeremy was horrified and couldn't move at first. He felt as though time stood still and that every detail of the event seemed vivid—the struggling cat, the motor oil sloshing over the cat and down his mouth, the teenager's laughing. He then turned and began to run back home, rushing into his bedroom and closing the door. He buried his head in his pillow and tried not to think about what he had just seen.

History of companion animals: Jeremy and his parents live with a cat who has been with the family since Jeremy was a baby.

Self-presentation: He readily talks about the incident and seems to need to vent. His affect is subdued.

Name: Adrian
Age: 10
Gender: Male
Ethnicity: Hispanic

Referral: Adrian was referred by juvenile's probation officer who has requested an assessment and possible recommendation to a diversion program. Adrian was involved in an incident involving abuse and death of a kitten and has been assigned to juvenile court.

Social and educational background: Adrian's parents work full-time at a local factory. Adrian's older sister, age 14, takes care of him after school, until mother returns at 8 p.m. The family owns its own home in a largely Hispanic lower-middle-class neighborhood. Adrian is an average student in the 4th grade and enjoys being at school with his friends. There is no complaint of unruly behavior from the school.

Precipitating events: Along with a friend of his, Adrian tried to drown a kitten in a bucket of water and then threw the kitten into a yard where it was killed by dogs. There is no further information about what the occasion of this act was.

History of companion animals: The family currently has a mixed-breed Alsatian dog. Another dog that they had from Adrian's early childhood died of natural causes two years ago.

Self-presentation: Adrian is big for his age. He is polite and cooperative in the initial interview. He does not understand the gravity of the situation.

Name: Martin
Age: 11
Gender: Male
Ethnicity: Caucasian

Referral: Juvenile court referred Martin for counseling. The police arrested him for animal abuse with three other boys. Martin and one of the other boys are 11 years old; two of the other boys are 13. The boys, who were riding their bikes, encountered a neighborhood cat sunning himself on the front steps of his house. At the suggestion of one of the older boys, they stopped and got off their bikes. One of the older boys approached the cat from the rear, grabbed him, and held the cat in the air. The other older boy took the cat and threw him into his empty backpack. They tossed the back-pack back and forth, and then one of them dropped the pack and began kicking it like a soccer ball. The cat was severely injured and died as a result of his injuries.

Social and educational background: Martin is in the 6 grade and is an average student. He has not had problems in school and no previous problems with juvenile authorities. He and the other 11-year-old involved in the incident are classmates. The older boys are poor students and have been in trouble for stealing, disrupting class, and bullying behavior.

Martin's family consists of his mother, father, and three older sisters. Mother describes Martin as difficult to manage as an infant and as a child easily bored and hot-tempered. Her husband was physically abusive to her in the past (damaged her retina with a beer bottle) and one assault with a gun. Father is an alcoholic and user of marijuana and cocaine.

Precipitating events: Martin maintained that grabbing the cat was not his idea and that he did not know the older boys were planning anything of that nature. Upon further questioning, he did acknowledge that he had heard from classmates that the older boys had "hurt animals" on a number of occasions. He admitted that he did participate in tossing the cat around but that he did not think that would really hurt the cat.

History of animal companions: The family currently has a 9-year-old dog. Reportedly, Martin has a good relationship with his dog and expresses fondness for her. There is no history of other cruelty to animals.

Self-presentation: Martin is initially talkative and relates well. However, he becomes defensive and then reticent when confronted with the incident. He said, "You can drop cats from something high and they always land on their feet." Martin said that he did not kick the backpack. When asked why he did not try to stop the other boys he just shook his head, not responding verbally. Martin said he was sorry that the cat was hurt, although he really does not like cats that much because they are "sneaky."

Name: Davie
Age: 11
Gender: Male
Ethnicity: Caucasian

Referral: Davie found a cat in his backyard eating his dog's food and hit it over the head with a shovel, killing it. Juvenile Justice found Davie guilty of cruelty to animals and deferred his possible removal from the home and placement in a detention center based on his compliance with a referral to this provider for AniCare treatment.

Social and educational background: Davie lives in a medium-sized city of 300,000 people in a neighborhood where there are people selling drugs and children are often unsupervised. His mother was addicted to drugs and gave Davie up to the care of his maternal grandmother. Davie was born with fetal alcohol syndrome and cocaine in his system. Both his biological parents have been in and out of jail. He has a biological brother who is one year younger and an uncle (who he considers his brother) who is 10 years older. There is a family dog who is 3 years old. Davie is in special education classes and enjoys drawing and math. He has a difficult time with reading and comprehension.

Precipitating events: Davie was shamed and ostracized by some older neighborhood boys earlier in the day, and there is a history of his aggressively acting out when made to feel inferior due to his thick glasses and special education needs. It is also uncertain what role, if any, his in utero drug exposure may have, but he also has seizures that are believed to be related to that exposure. He is very protective of the family dog and stated he felt like the cat was in some way a threat to the dog (if only her food supply).

History of companion animals: Davie and his "mother" consider themselves animal lovers and rescued their family companion animal three years ago from a neighbor who no longer wanted her. She is a 3½-year-old German shepherd mix whom he cares for very much but whom "mother" claims Davie can be "inappropriate" with (meaning he has touched her private parts) and "tongue kissed" with her. He has a history of killing insects and one amphibian, and "mother" has told him that this is unacceptable behavior. She was shocked by the killing of the cat.

Self-presentation: Davie is very shy and small for his age. He wears glasses and has somewhat protruding eyes. He speaks only intermittently and has attentional and oppositional problems. He was judged informally to have below-average intelligence. He responds well to positive attention.

Name: George
Age: 13
Gender: Male
Ethnicity: Caucasian

Referral: George entered a shelter with three other boys and bludgeoned 18 cats to death. George was perplexed by his arrest and his requirement to undergo counseling, stating "They were only cats!" His sentiment that "they were only cats" was shared by his friends and family.

Social and educational background: Mother describes George as difficult to manage as an infant and as a child easily bored and hot-tempered. Her husband was physically abusive to her in the past (damaged her retina with a beer bottle) and once assaulted her with a gun. Father is an alcoholic and user of marijuana and cocaine.

George is an average student in the 7th grade. He is uninterested in school or studies.

Precipitating events: George asserted that he and his friends wanted to "have some fun" to celebrate the beginning of summer vacation. They thought it would be "funny" to break into the local shelter and "knock some cats around."

History of companion animals: The family currently has a dog about whom George talks about with great relish, Sparkle. He said that sometimes Sparkle slept with him and that he would often take her on long walks. He recalled a time when he lost contact with Sparkle during one of their walks. George called for her repeatedly but she didn't respond. He went back home and enlisted the aid of his sister, and together they searched for Sparkle. After about two hours they finally found her; Sparkle had been caught in a steel-jaw leghold trap. In recalling this event, George displayed great feeling—he had tears in his eyes and found it difficult to talk through his emotions. He offered, "I felt so bad for her. Imagine what it was like to be caught like that and never know if someone was going to come and help you. I bet she wondered where I was and why I hadn't gotten there sooner."

Self-presentation: George is immediately verbally assertive, presenting his case against cats, and showing little respect for the authority of the therapist. Cats are "sneaky;" "you can't trust them." When asked how he imagined the cats felt that night he couldn't grasp the question. It was exceedingly difficult for George to put himself in the cats' position.

Name: Jason
Age: 14
Gender: Male
Ethnicity: African-American

Referral: Jason is currently in residential treatment for children with sexual trauma and sexual offender issues. His case manager requested treatment for his sexual behavior with animals.

Social and educational background: At age 5, Jason first came into care for severe sexual abuse against him by multiple perpetrators, both genders. He was placed in foster care at age 7 and had several placements before being adopted at age 10. While in one foster placement, he was given up due to aggressive behavior toward the foster mother, bumping up against her. He had "mutual consent contact" with another foster child and mutual masturbation and anal sex done on Jason. It is not clear if it was forced. He had counseling in his adoptive home but not directed specifically at his sexual behavior with animals.

Jason is capable of working at grade level—eighth grade. However, he often acts out in class, e.g., saying he is going to throw up. Other manipulative behaviors in school include lying.

Precipitating events: Jason injured a dog in the neighborhood during a sexual assault. He also occasionally scrapes his arm along a ledge until it bleeds.

History of companion animals: While still with his biological parents, he witnessed and was forced to participate in sexual abuse of an animal. While in foster care, he had sexual contact with animals. In one foster placement, he brought home a stray dog and slept in bed with it at night. It is unknown if he had sexual contact with the dog. There are also reports of rough handling (e.g., grabbing by neck) of a dog at one home, although, apparently, others at the home handled the dogs the same way.

Self-presentation: Jason is cooperative in the session and shows good verbal ability. His appearance is well kempt and his dress is stylish.

Name: Charles
Age: 15
Gender: Male
Ethnicity: African-American

Referral: Charles left his two pit bulls tied in the backyard unattended. One cannibalized the other and was eventually noticed by Charles' uncle, who provided for the remaining dog and he recovered. Juvenile Justice found Charles "involved" in cruelty to animals and referred him to counseling.

Social and educational background: Charles lives in a large city with his mother, who is addicted to crack. His father is currently in jail. He has one other younger sibling and his uncle lives nearby. He is a mediocre student and also works part-time at odd jobs.

Precipitating events: Charles received a minor injury from a gunshot by a boy in the neighborhood. Shortly thereafter, in an accident involving the dogs, the wound was reopened. Charles stayed in his room for three months, leaving the dogs uncared for in the backyard.

History of companion animals: Charles had rescued the two dogs two years ago when he found them abandoned. His knowledge of the needs of the dogs is very limited.

Self-presentation: Charles is a shy young man who appears depressed. When he does speak, he appears to be of average intelligence.

The following three cases are featured in the AniCare Child Demonstration DVD:

Name: Michael
Age: 9
Gender: Male
Ethnicity: Caucasian

Referral: Michael's parents brought him to counseling at the teacher's suggestion. He is impulsive in the classroom, often jumping up and hit/tapping other kids on the head. He seems easily frustrated by a variety of tasks—writing, sports, and artwork.

Name: Amanda
Age: 12
Gender: Female
Ethnicity: Caucasian

Referral: Amanda's mother called the school counselor when she saw Amanda treating their family cat roughly. On one occasion Amanda put the family cat in a dresser drawer and closed the drawer, leaving the room. The mother heard the cat's meows and released it. Another time, the mother observed Amanda dangling the cat out of the bedroom window.

The school counselor asked about the family. The mother explained those six months ago and the father had lost his job and has not been able to find work. He began drinking heavily. When he drinks, he becomes abusive, storming around the house, threatening anything that is in front of him. In fits of anger and yelling, he has threatened to kill Amanda's cat.

The school counselor recommended counseling for Amanda and for the family.

Name: Joel
Age: 16
Gender: Male
Ethnicity: African-American

Referral: Joel was arrested on animal abuse charges with two 19-year-old boys. Joel's parents are divorced; he lives with his mother and two younger sisters. Has infrequent contact with his father. He makes good grades in school, but tells his mother that he doesn't feel good about himself. Compared to the "in" kids at school, he doesn't feel cool.

The two older boys arrested with Joel are high school dropouts and live in the vicinity of Joel's house. The older boys frequently hang out at the school at the end of the school day.

Joel was walking home from school when he encountered the two older boys. According to Joel, they pressured him into going to a neighbor's house and stealing one of her rabbits from a hutch in the backyard. They then went to another neighbor's house and released his pit bull, which followed them to the field. They hung up the rabbit and encouraged the pit bull to kill him, which the dog did. Neighbors reported the incident to police, who investigated it, and arrested Joel. The older two boys are awaiting trial for felony charges. Joel, being underage, was adjudicated when terms of probation were set, including mandatory counseling.

5.6   Appendix F

5.6.1   Use of the *AniCare Child* Demonstration DVD

The DVD opens with a two-minute introduction that can be bypassed by clicking on "DVD Menu." Note that software for presentation of DVDs, such as Windows Media Player and RealPlayer, vary on how they designate such options and in the degree of flexibility they offer for fast-forwarding within a segment and for moving to segments at different levels.

The Main Menu has four headers:

I. What is the *AniCare Child* Model? (3 min)

II. Assessment (2 min)

Submenu

A. Assessment Interview with MICHAEL (see Appendix E: Supplemental Case Materials): Role-play showing use of the Animal-Related Experiences Inventory (8 min; see pp. 71–75) in context of an initial session

B. Assessment Factors. Use of the "Factors to consider in the assessment of juvenile animal abuse" (30 sec; see p. 9, Handbook) that supplements the ARE Inventory

C. Witnessing Animal Abuse (30 sec; see pp. 15–16).

III. Treatment. Introduction (30 sec)

Submenu

A. Self-management Skills: Problem-solving. Introduction (1 min). Role-play showing use of the SOLVE problem-solving technique with MICHAEL (8 min)

B. Self-management Skills: Projective Techniques. Introduction (90 sec). Demonstration of the Animals-at-Risk Thematic Apperception Test with AMANDA (first 9 of 17 min); crisis management demonstration (second 8 of 17 min) with AMANDA

C. Empathy Skills. Introduction (2 min 45 sec). Demonstration of Interactive Sequence Drawing technique with JOEL (34 min. 52 sec)

IV. Videos and Resources

Animals Aloud—classroom empathy exercise

Project Second Chance—youthful offender program with animal-assisted activity

5.7   Appendix G

5.7.1   Practitioner Exercises

The following exercises are intended as aids to therapists learning the AniCare approach. Each exercise is referenced in the main body of the text so you can try them while you go through the workbook.

If you would like personal feedback from a certified AniCare trainer, send the materials you produce from any or all of the exercises you complete to ken.shapiro@animalsandsociety.org. More formal and systematic consultation/supervision is also available.

1. Typology
The psychology of juvenile animal abuse takes many different forms. Pick 10 cases, supplementing those presented in the workbook, the Demonstration DVD, and the Supplemental Cases (Appendix E) with those available on www.pet-abuse.com. To gain access to the cases on the pet-abuse site, simply go to the Cruelty Database, register, search your state of residence, and read some of the recent cases posted. (To receive updates on cases of particular interest, sign up for them under Monitored Cases.) Develop your own typology of kinds of cases, think about the most fitting theoretical frame for formulating each (cognitive behavior, psychodynamic, attachment theory, family systems, etc.), and indicate likely diagnosis for each.

2. Factors to Consider...
Pick two cases from the ten you selected in Exercise 1. Using the categories in the Factors, provide a description of two of the cases. Use list, not narrative, form. For example, under the Psychodynamics/Motivations subsection, select those that apply to each case.

3. Demonstration Assessment Interview
After studying the Animal-Related Experiences Inventory and the Factors Considered...., view the "Assessment/Interview of Michael" (Demonstration DVD, Assessment submenu). Comment on the therapist's tone, style, rapport with client, working relation with client, structuring of interview, coverage of important areas of assessment, anything else that struck you about the therapist, and alternative ways of using the inventory. Focus on the therapist, not directly on the assessment of Michael. Note that the inventory is a screening device and that a full assessment interview might take more than one full session.

4. Empathy
Provide a critique of the use of the Interactive Drawing Technique ("Empathy Skills" [DVD, Treatment submenu] with Joel).

5. Self-Management
Provide a critique of the use of the SOLVE technique (pp. 43–46; "Self-Management Skills: Problem-Solving" (Demonstration DVD, Treatment submenu)) as an aid in

developing problem-solving and related self-management skills. Comment both on both the instrument itself and the therapist's use of it.

6. Animals-at-Risk Thematic Apperception Test

Pick one case from the 10 you selected in Exercise 1. Recruit a volunteer and have him or her read the case. Using standard instructions (p. 52), administer 4–5 of the A-TAT stimulus cards to the volunteer. Select those that you think would most likely solicit relevant themes for the case. Once the inquiry part of the assessment is completed, select a story and use it to work with the client on one of the interventions— accountability, empathy, or self-management. For example, for empathy, ask the volunteer to role-play the main character (human or nonhuman animal) in the story, or for self-management, ask the volunteer to provide alternative outcomes and evaluate them using SOLVE.

7. Assessment and Intervention Interviews

Conduct an assessment and an intervention interview with a juvenile. Arrange to use the same person to role-play each of the two interviews. Audiotape each interview. Interviews should be about 45 minutes.

To role-play the client, select someone you do not know well to avoid injecting your prior knowledge of his or her personality in your write-up. (Adults can role-play juveniles.) Provide the volunteer with a printout of one of the cases in Appendix E, Supplemental Cases. Instruct the volunteer to embroider on that description and to stay in role throughout the interview. Inform the volunteer of the purpose of the exercise, assure him or her of confidentiality, and provide debriefing following the interview as the material may be distressing.

The purpose of the *assessment* interview is to provide a picture of the person that can be used for diagnosis and as a guide to developing a treatment plan. Although the process can be therapeutic and certainly should not be harmful, it is not a therapeutic intervention. Cover enough ground in the interview to form an adequate picture of the client's difficulties. Use the "Animal-Related Experience Inventory and the Factors Considered..." as guides in a semi-structured interview, not as a checklist. Finally, based on your assessment of the client's needs, develop a treatment plan.

In a four- to five-page paper, provide an assessment of the client, including diagnostic impressions and treatment plans; provide critique of the assessment instruments. If you would like feedback on your interview and write-up, transcribe the interview and include with paper.

The purpose of the *intervention* interview is to think about the appropriate application of the various interventions in AniCare Child. For the interview, select an initial intervention related to accountability, identifying feelings, empathy development, or self-management. The purpose of the interview is to apply one or more of the interventions in the context of a free-flowing therapy session.

In a four- to five-page paper, provide an evaluation of the intervention(s)—your choice of specific interventions, your use of them, their impact on the client, and your opinion of the intervention(s) effectiveness, both in this case and generally for this population. If you would like feedback on your interview and write-up, transcribe the interview and include with paper.

References

Ainsworth, M. D. S., Blehar, M. C., Waters, E., & Wall, S. (1978). *Patterns of attachment: A psychological study of the strange situation*. Hillsdale, NJ: Lawrence Erlbaum Associates.

Alexander, J., Barton, C., Gordon, D., Grotpeter, J., Hansson, K., Harrison, R., et al. (1998). *Blueprints for violence prevention, book three: Functional family therapy*. Boulder: Center for the Study of Prevention of Violence.

Allen, K. (1996). Anger and hostility among married couples: Pet dogs as moderators of cardiovascular reactivity to stress. *Psychosomatic Medicine, 58*, 59–70.

Allen, K. (1998). Social interaction and cardiovascular reactivity within marriage: A focus on couples with and without pet cats and dogs. *Psychosomatic Medicine, 60*, 100.

Allen, K., & Blascovich, J. (1996). The value of service dogs for people with severe ambulatory difficulties. *Journal of the American Medical Association, 275*, 1001–1006.

Allen, K., Blascovich, J., Tomaka, J., & Kelsey, R. (1991). Presence of human friends and pet dogs as moderators of autonomic responses to stress in women. *Journal of Personality and Social Psychology, 61*, 582–589.

American Psychiatric Association (1987). *Diagnostic and statistical manual of mental disorders III-R*. Washington, DC: American Psychiatric Association.

American Psychiatric Association (1994). *Diagnostic and statistical manual of mental disorders IV*. Washington, DC: American Psychiatric Association.

Arluke, A. (1997). Interviewer guides used in cruelty research. *Anthrozoös, 10*, 180–182.

Ascione, F. R. (1992). Enhancing children's attitudes about the humane treatment of animals: Generalization to human-directed empathy. *Anthrozoös, 5*, 176–191.

Ascione, F. R. (1993). Children who are cruel to animals: A review of research and implications for developmental psychopathology. *Anthrozoös, 6*, 226–247.

Ascione, F. R. (1998). Battered women's reports of their partners' and their children's cruelty to animals. *Journal of Emotional Abuse, 1*, 119–133.

Ascione, F. R. (2000). What veterinarians need to know about the link between animal abuse and interpersonal violence. *Proceedings of the 137th annual meeting of the American Veterinary Medical Association* (CD-ROM records #316317), Salt Lake City, UT.

Ascione, F. R. (2001, September). Animal abuse and youth violence. In *Juvenile justice bulletin*. Rockville, MD: Office of Juvenile Justice and Delinquency Prevention (OJJDP).

Ascione, F. R. (2007). Emerging research on animal abuse as a risk factor for intimate partner violence. In K. Kendall-Tackett & S. Giacomoni (Eds.), *Intimate partner violence* (pp. 3-1–3-17). Kingston, NJ: Civic Research Institute.

Ascione, F. R., Kaufmann, M. E., & Brooks, S. M. (2000). Animal abuse and developmental psychopathology: Recent research, programmatic, and therapeutic issues and challenges for the future. In A. Fine (Ed.), *Handbook on animal-assisted therapy: Theoretical foundations and guidelines for practice* (pp. 325–354). New York: Academic Press.

Ascione, F. R., & Shapiro, K. (2009). People and animals, kindness and cruelty. *Journal of Social Issues, 65*, 565–589.

Ascione, F. R., Thompson, T. M., & Black, T. (1997). Childhood cruelty to animals: Assessing cruelty dimensions and motivations. *Anthrozös, 10*, 170–177.

Baker, D. G., Boat, B. W., Grinvalsky, H. T., & Geraciotti, T. D. (1998). Interpersonal trauma and animal-related experiences in female and male military veterans: Implications for program development. *Military Medicine, 163*, 20–25.

Baldry, A. C. (2003). Animal abuse and exposure to interparental violence in Italian youth. *Journal of Interpersonal Violence, 18*(3), 258–281.

Beck, A., Hunter, K., & Seraydarian, L. (1986). Use of animals in the rehabilitation of psychiatric inpatients. *Psychological Reports, 58*, 63–66.

Beck, A., & Katcher, A. (1984). A new look at pet-facilitated therapy. *Journal of the American Veterinary Medical Association, 184*, 414–421.

Beck, A., & Katcher, A. (1996). *Between pets and people: The importance of animal companionship*. West Lafayette: Purdue University Press.

Bickerstaff, G. (2003). *An exploration of animal abuse and animal abusers*. State University of New York, at Albany. Unpublished dissertation.

Boat, B. (1995). The relationship between violence to children and violence to animals: An ignored link? *Journal of Interpersonal Violence, 10*, 229–235.

Boat, B. (1999). Abuse of children and abuse of animals: Using the links to inform child assessment and protection. In F. R. Ascione & P. Arkow (Eds.), *Child abuse, domestic violence, and animal abuse: Linking the circles of compassion for prevention and intervention* (pp. 83–100). West Lafayette: Purdue University Press.

Bowlby, J. (1969). *Attachment and loss, Vol. 1: Attachment*. New York: Basic Books.

Bowlby, J. (1973). *Attachment and loss, Vol 2: Separation*. New York: Basic Books.

Bowlby, J. (1980). *Attachment and loss, Vol 3: Loss*. New York: Basic Books.

Bowlby, J. (1984). Violence in the family as a disorder of the attachment and caregiving systems. *The American Journal of Psychoanalysis, 44*, 9–27.

Bowlby, J. (1988). *A secure base*. New York: Basic Books.

Cavell, T. A. (2000). *Working with parents of aggressive children: A practitioner's guide*. Washington, DC: American Psychological Association.

Centers for Disease Control and Prevention, National Center for Injury Prevention and Control. (2010). Web-based Injury Statistics Query and Reporting System (WISQARS) [online]. Cited June 14, 2010, from www.cdc.gov/injury/wisqars/index.html

Christophersen, E. R. (1990). *Beyond discipline: Parenting that lasts a lifetime*. Kansas City, MO: Westport Publishers.

Christophersen, E. R., & Mortweet, S. L. (2001). *Treatments that work with children: Empirically supported strategies for managing childhood problems*. Washington, DC: American Psychological Association.

Cohen, J., Mannarino, A., & Deblinger, E. (2006). *Treating trauma and traumatic grief in children and adolescents*. New York: Guilford Press.

Coren, S. (2004). *How dogs think*. New York: Free Press.

Crowley-Robinson, P., Fenwick, D. C., & Blackshaw, J. K. (1996). A long-term study of elderly people in nursing homes with visiting and resident dogs. *Applied Animal Behavior Science, 47*, 137–148.

Cunningham, C., & MacFarlane, K. (1996). *When children abuse: Group treatment strategies for children with impulse control problems*. Brandon, VT: The Safer Society Press.

Degenhardt, B. (2004). *The statistical summary of offenders charged with crimes against companion animals: July 2001–July 2004*. Chicago: Chicago Police Department.

DeGue, S., & DiLillo, D. (2009). Is animal cruelty a "red flag" for family violence? *Journal of Interpersonal Violence, 24*, 1036–1056.

Deviney, E., Dickert, J., & Lockwood, R. (1983). The care of pets within child abusing families. *International Journal for the Study of Animal Problems, 4*, 321–329.

deZulueta, F. (1993). *From pain to violence*. Northvale, NJ: Jason Aronson.

Di Pellegrino, G., Fadiga, L., Fogassi, L., Gallese, V., & Rizzolatti, G. (1992). Understanding motor events: A neurophysiological study. *Experimental Brain Research, 91*, 176–180.

Dodge, K. A., & Coie, J. D. (1987). Social information processing factors in reactive and proactive aggression in children's peer groups. *Journal of Personality and Social Psychology, 53*, 1146–1158.

Dodge, K. A., & Crick, N. R. (1990). Social information-processing bases of aggressive behavior in children. *Personality and Social Psychology Bulletin, 16*, 8–22.

Eisenberg, N., & Strayer, J. (1987). Critical issues in the study of empathy. In N. Eisenberg & J. Strayer (Eds.), *Empathy and its development* (pp. 3–13). Cambridge: Cambridge University Press.

Ellis, A. (1986). Rational-emotive therapy. In I. L. Kutash & A. Wolf (Eds.), *Psychotherapist's casebook* (pp. 277–287). San Francisco: Jossey-Bass Publishers.

Eron, L. (1987). The development of aggressive behavior from the perspective of a developing behaviorism. *The American Psychologist, 42*, 435–442.

Feldman, J., & Kazdin, A. E. (1995). Parents management training for oppositional and conduct problem children. *Clinical Psychologist, 48*(4), 3–5.

Felthous, A. R., & Kellert, S. R. (1987). Childhood cruelty to animals and later aggression against people: A review. *The American Journal of Psychiatry, 144*, 710–717.

Fine, A. (2000). Animals and therapists: Incorporating animals in outpatient psychotherapy. In A. Fine (Ed.), *Handbook on animal-assisted therapy: Theoretical foundations and guidelines for practice* (pp. 179–208). New York: Academic Press.

Flynn, C. P. (1999). Exploring the link between corporal punishment and children's cruelty to animals. *Journal of Marriage and the Family, 61*, 971–981.

Flynn, C. P. (2000). Why family professionals can no longer ignore violence toward animals. *Family Relations, 49*, 87–95.

Fonagy, P., & Target, M. (1996). A contemporary psychoanalytical perspective: Psychodynamic developmental therapy. In E. D. Hibbs & P. S. Jensen (Eds.), *Psychosocial treatments for child and adolescent disorders: Empirically based strategies for clinical practice* (pp. 619–638). Washington, DC: American Psychological Association.

Forehand, R., & McMahon, R. J. (1981). *Helping the noncompliant child: A clinician's guide to parent training*. New York: Guilford Press.

Forgatch, M., & Patterson, G. (1989). *Parents and adolescents living together — Part 2: Family problem solving*. Eugene, OR: Castalia.

Frick, P. J., Lahey, B. B., Loeber, R., Tannenbaum, L., Van Horn, Y., Christ, M. A. G., et al. (1993). Oppositional defiant disorder and conduct disorder: A meta-analytic review of factors analyses and cross-validation in a clinic sample. *Clinical Psychology Review, 13*, 123–138.

Friedmann, E., & Lockwood, R. (1991). Validation and use of the animal thematic apperception test. *Anthrozoös, 4*(3), 174–183.

Garrity, T. F., & Stallones, L. (1998). Effects of pet contact. In C. C. Wilson & D. C. Turner (Eds.), *Companion animals in human health* (pp. 3–22). Thousand Islands, CA: Sage.

Goldstein, A. P. (1999). *Low-level aggression: First steps on the ladder to violence*. Champaign, IL: Research Press.

Gray, B. J. (1990). *Problem-solving for teens: An interactive approach to learning*. East Moline, IL: Lingua Systems.

Gupta, M. (2008). Functional links between intimate partner violence and animal abuse: Personality features and representations of aggression. *Society and Animals, 16*, 223–242.

Henggeler, S. W., Mihalic, S. F., Rone, L., Thomas, C., & Timmons-Mitchell, J. (1998). *Blueprints for violence prevention, book six: Multisystemic therapy*. Boulder, CO: Center for the Study and Prevention of Violence.

Henry, B. C. (2004). The relationship between animal cruelty, delinquency, and attitudes toward the treatment of animals. *Society and Animals, 12*(3), 185–207.

Henry, B, & Sanders, C. (2007). Bullying and animal abuse: Is there a connection? *Society and Animals, 15*, 107–126.

Hensley, C., Tallichet, E., & Dutkiewicz, E. L. (2009). Recurrent childhood animal cruelty: Is there a relationship to adult recurrent interpersonal violence. *Criminal Justice Review, 34*(2), 248–257.

Hilton, J. M., Anngela-Cole, L., & Wakita, J. (2010). A cross-cultural comparison of factors associated with school bullying in Japan and the United States. *The Family Journal, 18*, 413–422.

Holcomb, R., & Meacham, M. (1989). Effectiveness of an animal-assisted therapy program in an inpatient psychiatric unit. *Anthrozoös, 2*, 259–264.

Hunter, V. (1991). John Bowlby: An interview. *Psychoanalytic Review, 78*, 159–175.

Jory, B., & Randour, M. L. (1999). *The AniCare model of treatment for animal abuse*. Washington Grove, MD: Psychologists for the Ethical Treatment of Animals.

Karen, R. (1994). *Becoming attached*. New York: Warner.

Kazdin, A. E. (1985). *Treatment of antisocial behavior in children and adolescence*. Homewood, IL: Dorsey Press.

Kazdin, A. E. (1987). Treatment of antisocial behavior in children: Current status and future directions. *Psychology Bulletin, 102*, 187–203.

Kazdin, A. E. (1995). *Conduct disorder in childhood and adolescence* (2nd ed.). Thousand Oaks, CA: Sage.

Kazdin, A. E. (1996). Problem solving and parent management in treating aggressive and antisocial behavior. In E. D. Hibbs & P. S. Jensen (Eds.), *Psychosocial treatments for child and adolescent disorders: Empirically based strategies for clinical practice* (pp. 377–408). Washington, DC: American Psychological Association.

Kazdin, A. E., Bass, D., Siegel, T., & Thomas, C. (1989). Cognitive-behavioral therapy and relationship therapy in the treatment of children referred for antisocial behavior. *Journal of Consulting and Clinical Psychology, 57*, 522–535.

Kazdin, A. E., Siegel, T., & Bass, D. (1992). Cognitive problem solving skills training and parent management training in the treatment of antisocial behavior in children. *Journal of Consulting and Clinical Psychology, 60*, 733–747.

Kazdin, A. E., & Weisz, J. R. (1998). Identifying and developing empirically supported child and adolescent treatments. *Journal of Consulting and Clinical Psychology, 66*, 19–36.

Kellert, S. R., & Felthous, A. R. (1985). Childhood cruelty toward animals among criminals and noncriminals. *Human Relations, 38*, 1113–1129.

Kernberg, P. F., & Chazan, S. E. (1991). *Children with conduct disorders*. New York: Basic Books.

Kobak, R. (1999). The emotional dynamics of disruptions in attachment relationships: Implications for theory, research, and clinical intervention. In J. Cassidy & P. R. Shaver (Eds.), *Handbook of attachment: Theory, research and application* (pp. 21–43). New York: Guilford Press.

Lahey, B. B., Loeber, R. L., Quay, H. C., Frick, P. J., & Grimm, J. (1992). Oppositional defiant and conduct disorders: Issue to be resolved for DSM-IV. *Journal of the American Academy of Child and Adolescent Psychiatry, 31*, 43–56.

Levy, T. M., & Orlans, M. (1998). *Attachment, trauma, and healing*. Washington, DC: CWLA Press.

Lewchanin, S., & Zimmerman, E. (2000). *Clinical assessment of juvenile animal abuse*. Brunswick, ME: Biddle Publishing Company & Audenreed Press.

Lockwood, R. (1983). The influence of animals on social perception. In A. H. Katcher & A. M. Beck (Eds.), *New perspectives on our lives with companion animals* (pp. 64–71). Philadelphia: University of Pennsylvania Press.

Lockwood, R. (1985). The role of animals in our perception of people. *The Veterinary Clinics of North America. Small Animal Practice, 15*(2), 377–385.

Lockwood, R. (1998). *Factors in the assessment of dangerousness in perpetrators of animal abuse* (Unpublished report). Washington, DC: Humane Society of the United States.

Lockwood, R., & Hodge, G. R. (1998). The tangled web of animal abuse: The links between cruelty to animals and human violence. In R. Lockwood & F. R. Ascione (Eds.), *Cruelty to animals and interpersonal violence*. West Lafayette, IN: Purdue University Press.

Loeber, R. (1990). Development and risk factors in juvenile anti-social behavior and delinquency. *Clinical Psychology Review, 10*, 1–42.

Loeber, R. (1991). Antisocial behavior: More enduring than changeable? *Journal of the American Academy of Child and Adolescent Psychiatry, 30*, 393–397.

Loeber, R., Wung, P., Keenan, K., Giroux, B., Stouthamer-Loeber, M., Van Kammen, W. B., et al. (1993). Developmental pathways in disruptive child behavior. *Development and Psychopathology, 5*, 103–133.

Luke, C., Arluke, A., & Levin, J. (1997). *Cruelty to animals and other crimes: A study by the MSPCA and Northeastern University.* Boston: Massachusetts Society for the Prevention of Cruelty to Animals.

Main, M., & Goldwyn, R. (1984). Predicting rejection of her infants from mother's representation of her own experience: Implications for the abused-abusing intergenerational cycle. *International Journal of Child Abuse and Neglect, 8,* 203–217.

Main, M., & Solomon, J. (1986). Discovery of a disorganized/disoriented attachment pattern. In T. B. Brazelton & M. W. Yogman (Eds.), *Affective development in infancy* (pp. 95–124). Norwood, NJ: Ablex.

Main, M., & Solomon, J. (1990). Procedures for identifying infants as disorganized/disoriented during the Ainsworth Strange Situation. In M. Greenberg, D. Cicchetti, & E. M. Cummings (Eds.), *Attachment in the preschool years* (pp. 121–160). Chicago: University of Chicago Press.

Martin, F. E. (1998). Tales of transition: Self-narrative and direct scribing in exploring care leaving. *Child and Family Social Work, 3*(1), 1–12.

McMahon, P. J., & Forehand, R. (1984). Parent training for the noncompliant child: Treatment outcomes, generalizations, and adjunctive therapy procedures. In R. F. Dangel & A. Polster (Eds.), *Parent training: Foundations of research and practice* (pp. 298–328). New York: Guilford Press.

Melson, G. F. (2001). *Why the wild things are.* Cambridge: Harvard University Press.

Miller, K. S., & Knutson, J. R. (1997). Reports of severe physical punishment and exposure to animal abuse by inmates convicted of felonies and by university students. *Child Abuse & Neglect, 21,* 59–82.

Miner, N. (1999, Fall). 1997–1998 School shootings roundup. *The Latham Letter,* p. 11.

Moeller, T. G. (2001). *Youth aggression and violence: A psychological approach.* Mahwah, NJ: Lawrence Erlbaum Associates.

Moffitt, T. E. (1993). Adolescence-limited and lifecourse-persistent antisocial behavior: A developmental taxonomy. *Psychological Review, 100,* 674–701.

Murray, H. (1951). Uses of the thematic apperception test. *The American Journal of Psychiatry, 107,* 577–581.

Orlansky, K. (2000). *Improving the response to domestic violence in Montgomery County* (Report No. 2000-1). Rockville, MD: Office of Legislative Oversight.

Patterson, G. R., DeBaryshe, B. D., & Ramsey, E. (1989). A developmental perspective on antisocial behavior. *The American Psychologist, 44,* 329–335.

Pekarik, G., & Stephenson, L. A. (1988). Adult and child client differences in therapy dropout research. *Journal of Clinical Child Psychology, 17,* 316–321.

Perelle, I. B., & Granville, D. A. (1993). Assessment of the effectiveness of a pet facilitated therapy program in a nursing home setting. *Society and Animals, 1,* 1–100.

Poresky, R. H. (1990). The young children's empathy measure: Reliability, validity and effects of companion animal bonding. *Psychological Reports, 66,* 931–936.

Poresky, R. H. (1996). Companion animals and other factors affecting young children's development. *Anthrozös, 9,* 159–168.

Risley-Curtiss, C. (2010). Social work practitioners and the human-companion animal bond: A national survey. *Social Work, 55,* 38–46.

Roberts, G. E. (1982). *Roberts' apperception test for children.* Torrance, CA: Western Psychological Services.

Robins, L. N. (1991). Conduct disorder. *Journal of Child Psychology and Psychiatry, 32,* 193–212.

Rutter, M., & Giller, H. (1983). Clinical practice of child psychiatry: A survey. *Journal of the American Academy of Child Psychiatry, 22,* 573–579.

Sable, P. (2000). *Attachment and adult psychotherapy.* Northvale, NJ: Jason Aronson.

Sanders, M. R., & Dadds, M. R. (1993). *Behavioral family intervention.* Needham Heights, MA: Allyn & Bacon.

Schachar, R., & Wachsmuth, R. (1990). Oppositional disorder in children: A validation study comparing conduct disorder, oppositional disorder and normal control children. *Journal of Psychology and Psychiatry, 31,* 1089–1102.

Schore, A. (2003). Early relational trauma, disorganized attachment, and the development of a predisposition to violence. In M. F. Solomon & D. J. Siegel (Eds.), *Healing trauma* (pp. 107–167). New York: W. W. Norton.

Schore, A. (2004). *Affect regulation and the repair of the self.* New York: Norton.

Scott, S. (1997). *Peer pressure reversal: An adult guide to developing a responsible child* (2nd ed.). Amherst, MA: HRD Press.

Serketich, W. J., & Dumas, J. E. (1996). The effectiveness of behavioral parent training to modify antisocial behavior in children: A meta analysis. *Behavior Therapy, 27,* 171–186.

Shapiro, K. J. (1990). The pedagogy of learning and unlearning empathy. *Phenomenology and Pedagogy, 8,* 42–48.

Siegel, D. J. (2003). An interpersonal neurobiology of psychotherapy: The developing mind and the resolution of trauma. In M. F. Solomon & D. J. Siegel (Eds.), *Healing trauma* (pp. 1–56). New York: W. W. Norton.

Simmons, A. C., & Lehmann, P. (2007). Exploring the link between pet abuse and controlling behaviors in violent relationships. *Journal of Interpersonal Violence, 22*(9), 1211–1222.

Simpson, J. A., & Rholes, W. S. (1998). *Attachment theory and close relationships.* New York: Guilford.

Tallichet, S. E., & Hensley, C. (2004). Exploring the link between recurrent acts of childhood and adolescent animal cruelty and subsequent violent crime. *Criminal Justice Review, 29,* 304–316.

Thomas, K., & Gullone, E. (2006). An investigation into the association between the witnessing of animal abuse adn adolescents' behavior toward animals. *Society and Animals, 14, 3,* 221–243.

Toby, J. (1995). The schools. In J. Q. Wilson & J. Petersilia (Eds.), *Crime* (pp. 141–170). San Francisco: Institute for Contemporary Studies Press.

Tyrrell, C., Dozier, M., Teague, G., & Fallot, R. (1999). Effective treatment relationships for persons with serious psychiatric disorders. *Journal of Consulting and Clinical Psychology, 67,* 725–733.

Vaughn, M. G., Fu, Q., DeLisi, M., Beaver, K., Perron, B., Terrell, K., et al. (2009). Correlates of cruelty to animals in the United States: results from the National Epidemiologic Survey on Alcohol and Related Conditions. *Journal of Psychiatric Research, 43,* 1213–1218.

Verlinden, S., Hersen, M., & Thomas, J. (2000). Risk factors in school shootings. *Clinical Psychology Review, 20,* 1, 3–56.

Vitiello, B., & Jensen, P. (1995). Disruptive behavior disorders. In H. I. Kaplan & B. J. Sadock (Eds.), *Comprehensive textbook of psychiatry* (6th ed., pp. 2311–2319). Baltimore: Williams & Wilkins.

Walton-Moss, B. J., Manganello, J., Frye, V., & Campbell, J. (2005). Risk factors for intimate partner violence and associated injury among urban women. *Journal of Community Health, 30*(5), 377–389.

Webster-Stratton, C. (1989). Systematic comparison of consumer satisfaction of three cost-effective parent training programs for conduct problem children. *Behavior Therapy, 20,* 103–115.

Webster-Stratton, C. (1996). Early intervention with videotape modeling: Programs for families of children with oppositional defiant disorder or conduct disorder. In E. D. Hibbs & P. S. Jensen (Eds.), *Psychosocial treatments for child and adolescent disorders: Empirically based strategies for clinical practice* (pp. 435–474). Washington, DC: American Psychological Association.

Webster-Stratton, C., & Hammond, M. (1997). Treating children with early-onset conduct problems: A comparison of child and parent training interventions. **Journal of Consulting and Clinical Psychology,** 65, 93–109.